DIFFERENT
STROKES

DIFFERENT STROKES

*An Intimate Memoir for
Stroke Survivors, Families,
and Caregivers*

STEVEN BOORSTEIN
FOREWORD BY JOHN NEWCOMBE
INTRODUCTION BY JIE MAO, MD

SKYHORSE PUBLISHING

Skyhorse Publishing books may be purchased in bulk at special discounts for sales promotion, corporate gifts, fund-raising, or educational purposes. Special editions can also be created to specifications. For details, contact the Special Sales Department, Skyhorse Publishing, or info@skyhorsepublishing.com.

Skyhorse® and Skyhorse Publishing® are registered trademarks of Skyhorse Publishing, Inc.®, a Delaware corporation.

www.skyhorsepublishing.com

10 9 8 7 6 5 4 3 2 1

Library of Congress Cataloging-in-Publication Data is available on file.
ISBN: 978-1-61608-471-4

NOTE: This book is not intended as a substitute for the medical advice of physicians. The reader should regularly consult a physician in matters relating to his/her health and particularly with respect to exercises and physical therapy.

Although the author and publisher have made every effort to ensure that the information in this book was correct at press time, the author and publisher do not assume and hereby disclaim any liability to any party for any loss, damage, or disruption caused by errors or omissions, whether such errors or omissions result from negligence, accident, or any other cause.

Printed in the United States of America

To my wife Barbara — my Florence Nightingale — and my sons Ben and Bryan. I would not be where I am today without their love and constant support.

I would also like to acknowledge my fourteen new friends and stroke survivors, as well as their spouses and partners, for sharing their stroke recovery stories with me.

CONTENTS

viii • DIFFERENT STROKES

INTRODUCTION BY DR. JIE MAO

In my line of work, I see numerous stroke victims. Katelyn is one example. Katelyn was admitted to the Emergency Room with a very bad sore throat. She'd had tonsillitis before, but this time the pain was particularly bad. She was coughing up blood, sometimes a whole cup at a time. Her ENT doctor suspected an infected blood vessel; a subsequent CT angiogram confirmed a *pseudoaneurysm*— a false aneurysm or bruise from a leaking hole in an artery—actively bleeding next to her right-side tonsil. Surgery was considered, but would have been dangerous. The amount of bleeding would have most likely hampered our visualization during surgery. Any attempt at clamping off that false aneurysm may have been futile, and could have resulted in damage to other surrounding structures such as the main carotid artery. I was called in to perform a catheter-directed angiogram, with intention to treat—meaning to embolize, or plug up, the false aneurysm from the inside. What we found was jaw-dropping.

Katelyn's right-sided middle cerebral artery, which supplied blood to half of the right side of her brain, was completely blocked! The tonsil infection had weakened her carotid artery, and had caused her to sustain a massive stroke. A physical exam performed immediately on the table confirmed complete left-sided hemiplegia (total paralysis) and an inability to speak. This lively, walking, talking nineteen-year-old girl with full potential was now looking at severe, permanent, life-threatening disabilities. Eight hours into what was an intense, adrenaline-pumping procedure, Katelyn's bleeding pseudoaneurysm was plugged up, and her artery was "opened" to the best of my ability.

Stroke happens to people in all walks of life. It affects the young and the old, and does not discriminate based on gender or race. Nearly 800,000 Americans are expected to have a stroke in 2011, increased from the 600,000 in 2005; that means, on average, a stroke occurs every 40 seconds in the United States. Stroke kills more than 137,000 people a year, and is the No. 3 cause of death behind heart disease and cancer. Someone dies of stroke roughly every 4 minutes. About 40 percent of stroke deaths occur in males and 60 percent in females. African Americans are more likely to be affected than white Americans.

Of those who survive a stroke, disabilities vary widely, depending on the size and location of the stroke. While medical procedures can be lifesaving, they do not address the emotional and physical challenges each stroke survivor faces after the attack. It is the ensuing months and years of rehabilitation, frustration, and heartwarming successes that truly mark the resilience and heroism of a stroke survivor.

Katelyn did recover. Her left arm still has deficits, but she has regained full function of her left leg and hand. Some people attribute this remarkable recovery to the fact that the stroke happened while she was on the angiographic table and that no time was wasted between the event and the treatment. Others attribute it to the fact that she's young and her brain is malleable. I believe it is due to her unrelenting willpower, positivity, and perseverance. One story, one life.

Different Strokes has something for everyone. It is touching, revealing, questioning, and inspiring. Steve's book tells his story and the stories of fourteen other survivors, along with six of their spouses. It provides a rare and precious glimpse into life after stroke for families and loved ones. Steve and his "survivors" put it all out there as they share the emotions and the realities of the young and old, the fit and sick—and the just plain unlucky. His emotional rollercoaster ride is always real, often funny, and even provocative. Steve dives headfirst into the heart and mind of a stroke survivor, and the experience that changes the lives of all those touched by it.

FOREWORD BY JOHN NEWCOMBE

Steve Boorstein has written an excellent personal and emotional account of his experience dealing with the aftermath of having a stroke.

My own episode occurred in 2003, when a small blood vessel on the left side of my brain started to bleed. Fortunately for me it sealed off and the damage was limited; I couldn't write for four months, and temporarily lost some of the feeling in my right foot and lower lip.

A year later I decided to write a book about my experience. As I researched the facts about strokes and the number of people of all ages who have experienced them, I realized that the general public does not have much knowledge about these "brain attacks." For years we have been given great insights into the workings of our hearts, but for some reason the thought of something going wrong with our brain is too scary to contemplate. Steve does an excellent job of conveying this through his poignant and humorous prose.

The fact is that many of these brain attacks are avoidable. Simply keeping an eye on your blood pressure, cholesterol, eating and drinking habits, and stress levels will help avoid the chances of one of these attacks. Reduce or give up smoking. Learn to breathe deeply and walk away from stressful situations.

The one area I am not convinced about is the low level of cholesterol that doctors in the United States and Australia are trying to bring us all down to. "Good" cholesterol is necessary for a number of important bodily functions.

Following my stroke, I was talked into taking 10 mg of

Lipitor every day, as my cholesterol was too high. Lipitor belongs to a class of drugs called statins, which dilute cholesterol but also attack the regeneration of our muscle tissues. After about six months I started getting strange pains throughout my body which I had never experienced before. About eighteen months later, my whole back went into an unbelievably painful spasm that took my kinesiologist five days of constant treatment to fix.

As soon as I had the attack I went off Lipitor and have experienced no muscle problems since. Two years ago my doctor talked me into taking 5 mg of another statin drug. The next morning I experienced five two-minute attacks of dizziness and stomach upset. So, for me, that was it for statins; and today I try to control cholesterol through diet and exercise. In Europe the doctors are not nearly so fanatic about low levels of cholesterol. (As an aside, my research revealed that the top-selling statin drug is worth $12 billion a year to the company that sells it. That can buy you a great amount of marketing and lobbying!)

After my book, *No One's Indestructible,* came out in Australia, I had many people come up to me in the street and say how much they had enjoyed it, and had given it to their spouse as a gift.

Steve's book will not only help people avoid a stroke, it is a must-read for those who have had an attack and for their friends and families. It's very brave to write about your innermost feelings, especially after your body has experienced an attack you wouldn't wish on your worst enemy.

Congratulations, Steve, and good luck. May I suggest you use this opportunity to fix any technical weakness you might have had in your tennis game?

–John Newcombe
Wimbledon Champion

INTRODUCTION

This book is about stroke. Not a tennis stroke—although tennis is a recurring theme. It is about the medical kind of stroke: an interruption of the blood supply to the brain. More specifically, it is about recovering from stroke, inspiration, and the life changes that result from this experience. I hope you'll find my book as entertaining as it is informative. It is addressed to all those who have suffered a stroke; to their partners, families, friends, and caregivers; and to all those who might wish to prevent stroke—or just read a compelling story.

Stroke is the third-leading cause of death in America, and for the "lucky" stroke victims who don't die, about half will spend the rest of their lives trying to recover. Most of these people will be changed forever—often in a good way. Fantastic as it may seem, many of those who have survived a stroke, regardless of their deficits and disabilities, would not give it back, even if they could. I am one of them.

I wrote this book because I had to, and because I wanted to do my part to help dispel the myth that strokes only happen to people in poor health. I represent a growing number of "healthy" people to have suffered a stroke not from plaque, illness, obesity, hypertension, poor eating habits, or smoking, but from a "typical" accident that eventually resulted in a stroke: an accident that could happen to anyone. Such an accident happened to me, when I was struck by a "hit and run" snowboarder while skiing. I've divided the book into three parts. In Part One, I'll describe my life before the stroke: my career as "The Clothing Doctor," an appearance on *The View*, rollerblading through the streets of London, learning the inner workings of bodysurfing, and moving to the mountains of Colorado at age fifty-three. I'll also describe the events that led to my stroke, my treatment, and its aftermath—when I awoke to find that I couldn't pick up an almond or tie my shoes—or even remember how to tie my shoes.

Fifty percent of strokes result in one-sided paralysis, my own included. People have certainly suffered more severe strokes than mine. But like all stroke survivors, I had to cope with despair and depression. I stayed the course of rehabilitation and worked my ass off to get better. I determined I would use some unconventional methods to regain my physical and cognitive abilities, and these led to the discoveries and life-changing insights that fed my recovery. I experienced the depression and disruption that accompany stroke, but I rose to become healthy again. I know that my experiences can help guide and comfort other survivors and their loved ones. My physical and occupational therapists told me repeatedly that my first year of recovery was an inspiration and an experience that should be shared with all stroke survivors, families of survivors, and rehabilitation therapists throughout the medical field. I'm sure my recovery and struggles will ring true to many survivors, and I hope my insights and somewhat unorthodox practices will deliver many inspiring and entertaining moments to help you through your personal hell, whatever that may be. However, as inspiring and entertaining as my story may be, we know that different folks have different strokes. They are in here too: I honor and deeply respect the twenty incredible survivors and spouses I interviewed for Part Two—some of whom are much worse off than me. There are few ailments more personal than stroke. These people put it all out there to tell their story. They welcomed me into many private places, without airs or preamble, and were willing to describe such experiences as:

- Sex after stroke
- How stroke affects relationships with children
- Life and personality changes—personally and professionally

Together, we hope to touch the heart and soul of every survivor, family member, and caregiver. In addition to my own story and that of the interviewees, in Part Three I have assembled a section of suggested exercises to aid in recovery; a glossary of medical terms and abbreviations pertinent to stroke; and a list of resources I and countless other stroke survivors have found helpful—and I hope you will too.

So here we go. I wish you the fortitude to persevere and the grace to benefit from your struggles as you or your loved one copes with the aftermath of stroke.

Steve Boorstein

PART ONE

MY STORY

Chapter 1

TIAs (APRIL 2, 2008)

I was sitting on the couch in my den, watching TV and playing guitar, when I got a severe headache, followed by tingling and numbness in my left shoulder, arm, and hand. I'd
had a history of migraines, which had grown worse after my
family and I moved to Boulder, Colorado, where we now live
in the foothills at an altitude of 6,500 feet. This felt different
to me from a classic migraine. It was very painful, but I did not
get the "aura" and blurriness that accompanies my migraines.
I figured that the tingling was a result of a shoulder dislocation
I had suffered during a freak ski accident three months before,
or maybe a pinched nerve.

The headache came on fast and furious, but subsided in
about fifteen minutes, which was also odd, as most migraines
last a few hours and then hang around for a day. The tingling lingered a bit longer than the headache, but I didn't
give it much more thought. I called a doctor friend who knew
about my ski accident and subsequent rehabilitation, to ask
him about my symptoms. We talked about the shoulder,
nerves, the numbness, the headaches, and even about stroke.
He steered the conversation away from stroke, since headache
is not always one of the typical symptoms and I did not have
any of the other telltale signs of stroke, such as face distortion,
disorientation, or slurred speech.

Barb and I were invited to a party that night, and I intended to go. After a lifetime of migraines I'd learned to cope
with the pain and had decided years before not to let these
things run or ruin my life. Back in sixth grade I'd wake up for

school with the aura and the pain, and I'd spend full days in bed, taking Darvon to help me sleep until the worst of the pain had subsided. But at forty-five, when I scored scalped third-row tickets for Paul McCartney and got a severe migraine one hour before the concert, I went anyway. "The show must go on," as they say. I had developed a high threshold for pain.

By the time I showered and dressed I felt fine. On the way to the party, I got another headache, again without the aura. My left shoulder and arm tingled and started going numb. It lasted a bit longer than the first episode. I took a Tylenol so I could dance and enjoy myself. I also drank a glass of wine. I started chatting with friends as the pain and tingling subsided, and proceeded to dance my ass off for the next few hours.

The following morning I ran some errands and then spent a few hours catching up on business. That afternoon I went to the acupuncturist, thinking that some well-placed needles might help what I assumed was a pinched nerve in my shoulder. The next day my shoulder felt fine, with no numbness. I figured that must have been it.

The following day I drove to Denver to pick up some custom packaging for shipping orders from our online store. After loading the boxes into the trunk, I hopped in the car and headed back to Boulder, typically a forty-minute drive. Just as I got in the car, the headache and the numbness on the left side returned. I started whacking that arm with my fist in disgust to "wake it up," but it didn't help. I tried to rethink the whole process, reasoning still that the tingling stemmed from the dislocation and damaged nerves. I must have pinched the nerve again loading the boxes. I was a healthy guy, very physical; I had no shortness of breath, no facial distortion. I shook off my puzzlement and steered my way back onto the highway toward Boulder.

This time, after the numbness went away, I started to experience some slight disorientation, and before I knew it, I had missed the exit for 36W and found myself heading west on 70 toward Golden and Vail. I got off in Golden and took 93S back to Boulder in a roundabout manner. It took about an hour and a half to find my way home, which was very strange given that I'd driven the same route many times when coming back from skiing.

I sat on the couch in the den and strummed my guitar. I started feeling badly, more than just odd. Another headache came on, and this time my arm went limp and I felt even more disoriented. My wife, Barb, got home a few minutes later, and I told her straightaway that I needed to go to the emergency room. We headed for the Broadway branch of Boulder Community Hospital, which was closest to our home. I called my doctor friend to see if he was working at the ER that day. He was on duty, but at the hospital's other location.

What I was experiencing was foreign, and it made me feel very vulnerable. I moaned and swayed in the passenger seat, finding comfort in the rhythm of the drive. What could be happening?

Months earlier, I had just returned to Boulder with Barb and my younger son Ben after ten fantastic days of sun, sand, and body surfing in San Pancho, Mexico. We were eagerly awaiting the visit of our older son, Bryan, over the Christmas vacation. The snow was coming down hard in Boulder and harder up in the mountains, which was a shock to our systems after the warmth of the past ten days. Nevertheless—as is the custom for skiers and outdoorsy people when the snow is dumping—Ben and I decided to go to Vail for a few days. We got up early and were on the slopes by eleven. We skied a few runs in hard-falling snow and then headed for the other side of the mountain.

On the way down to the lifts at Mid Vail, with Ben up the hill and out of sight, an unseen skier or snowboarder slammed into me—HARD. I awoke maybe thirty seconds later with a sinking feeling and a lot of pain. Both my skis had released and my poles rolled down the hill, but my helmet was still on my head in one piece. My goggles were cracked, and I had a gash on my nose. I also had a large black spot moving across my left eye and obscuring my vision. I knew these spots from past experience; they are called "floaters."

I'd fallen before, but this time felt different. I was whacked out. I could see Ben standing next to me, asking what happened and if I was okay. I tried to get up, but could not. I felt my left shoulder and knew something was very wrong. After a few moans and some dark moments trying to assess my condition, I realized that I needed a ski patrol and a toboggan ride down the mountain—my first in a lifetime of skiing. Twenty-one-year-old Ben was a bit freaked, as he'd never seen me hurt, but was very helpful. A skier on the lift above us yelled down to see if I needed help, and he summoned a ski patrol.

In a few very painful minutes I was preliminarily diagnosed with a dislocated shoulder and a possible concussion. Ben gathered my skis, poles, and helmet, and then helped the ski patrol secure my shoulder in a sling and roll me onto the toboggan. Every turn and bump of the ride down caused extreme pain and discomfort. I spoke gently to myself and tried to get lost in the rhythm and roll of the ride. I replayed the fiasco in my mind over and over as I tried to comprehend what had happened.

I'd skied my whole life and was quite accomplished. I may have had one close brush with another skier in forty-five years, but had never been hit. The person who hit me did not stop. This was a new phenomenon, as fallen skiers had started suing the people who hit them. Hence there had been a growing trend for skiers and boarders—mostly young people—to "hit and run," rather than stop and take responsibility. I'd read about it in the Boulder newspapers, so I knew that it happened, and I skied at my own risk. Still, I was shocked someone would run me down and not stop to help.

I heard the ski patrol assuring me that we'd be there in just a few minutes. We reached the bottom and the emergency team lifted the toboggan like a gurney. I was loaded, gingerly, into a Suburban at the base of the mountain, then driven to the Emergency Room at Vail Hospital, where I was efficiently rolled off the toboggan and onto a hospital examining table.

The ER personnel needed to remove my four layers of clothing for the exam and X-rays. I asked that they not cut off the clothing, as it had cost me hundreds of dollars. They obeyed, but warned me that the pain of removing the parka, ski sweater, shirt, and insulated undershirt over my shoulder would be intense. I told them to try; they were right, it hurt. I was ushered into an examining room, where they left me for what felt like far too long. I answered the nurse's typical questions, describing the hit, the fall, the result, and my current physical and mental condition.

The doctor finally came in. He said that he was going to "gently" pop my shoulder back in, without medication, and then send me for X-rays. During his exam, he realized that I probably had some broken ribs as well. For any of you who have endured the resetting of a dislocated shoulder, you know how painful it is. For the rest of you—I hope you never find out. I went from incredible pain during the resetting to a somewhat relaxed state of pain and discomfort once my shoulder was back where it belonged.

They took the X-rays, told me that my shoulder was properly relocated but that I had hairline cracks in four ribs on my right side. They gave me some instructions and a prescription for Vicodin, and sent me off to the rehabilitation center for some physical therapy exercises and advice. The physical therapist put me in a new sling, and I left the hospital on my own two feet, feeling spent and deeply depressed. Ben, a true champ, gently steered me to our car, helped buckle me into the front seat, and then drove us back to our condo in Vail. I took the Vicodin and waited for it to take effect.

Between the dislocated shoulder, the accompanying torn ligaments on my left side, and the cracked ribs on the right side, I felt extremely fragile. Breathing became very painful. I met with a local orthopedist later in the week for further examination.

My orthopedist back east, who had treated me through the years for various tennis injuries, always maintained that it was best to keep moving, barring any broken bones. In his opinion it was perfectly fine to use—but not to abuse—sprained or twisted joints, and I tried to follow that advice when possible. The Boulder orthopedist assured me that the shoulder was a clean dislocation, and that both it and the torn ligaments should heal in a few months with the requisite physical therapy. My ribs, on the other hand, would be extremely painful and difficult to heal. There was nothing to do for them, other than rest, for five to six weeks.

He was right. Breathing, moving, and sleeping became the bane of my life, and it would be almost five weeks before I could sleep on either side or on my back. I slept sitting up during that whole period.

What Had Been Happening in My Den: TIAs (Transient Ischemic Attacks)

It turned out that I had experienced a number of TIAs (transient ischemic attacks) over the past week. A TIA is a "warning stroke" or "mini-stroke" that produces stroke-like symptoms but no lasting damage. Recognizing and treating TIAs can reduce the risk of a major stroke. Most strokes are not preceded by TIAs, but a person who's had one or more attacks is more likely to have a stroke than someone of the same age and sex who hasn't. In fact, of the people who've had one or more TIAs, more than one-third will later have a stroke.

TIAs are more important in predicting *if* a stroke will occur than *when* one will occur. They can happen days, weeks, or even months before a major stroke. In about half the cases, the stroke occurs within one year of the TIA.

TIAs are caused when a blood clot or plaque temporarily clogs an artery, and part of the brain doesn't get the blood it needs. The symptoms occur rapidly and last a relatively short time, hence the diminishing tingling in my left arm. Most TIAs last less than five minutes. The average is about one minute. Unlike stroke, when a TIA is over, the injury to the brain is so small that there usually isn't any long-term effect. However, there may be cumulative effects of many TIAs if left untreated.

Of course, on that fateful day I knew none of this, and felt only fear and confusion. I still believed that whatever was happening must be a minor side effect of my recent skiing accident. I had a lot to learn.

Chapter 2

REHABILITATION AND GETTING BACK ON THE SLOPES: WEEK BEFORE THE STROKE

I hit a few tennis balls during the rib rehab to loosen me up, with some accompanying pain and discomfort. But my ribs finally healed, returning to normal, and I never looked back. The large black floater in my left eye that I sustained during the fall was another story. It never did go away—another battle scar, I guess. After many months my shoulder improved, but never fully healed, so I lost most of my range of motion. I used to be able to scratch my own back and was limber enough to reach around and "lock" hands with my other arm, but now could not even get my left arm halfway up my back. I couldn't even comfortably rest my left arm out the window while driving.

I'd always believed that after the requisite amount of rehab—or after a few days for lesser injuries—the return to normalcy is up to the individual. With my other injuries, from twisted ankles to knee sprains, I always returned to sports and movement as soon as humanly possible, even if it meant considerable discomfort. This time I began hitting tennis balls, though I couldn't toss the ball up for a proper serve, since that required the use of my left arm.

That left skiing. I decided to test my physical and emotional condition by skiing Eldora, our "local" ski resort thirty minutes up Boulder Canyon, just outside of town. Though I kept a positive attitude, I wrestled with the fear of being hit again. Every pole plant and turn jarred the shoulder, causing some acute—but passing—pain. Since it felt promising, I stepped up the speed, committed to my turns, and began to really feel it. I loved skiing Eldora, even though it was a small resort compared to Breckenridge or Vail. Most of the people came from Boulder and surrounding towns, so there was a decent chance that you'd meet someone on the lift who could become a friend or future ski partner.

At one point I hit a sizable bump at high speed, which caused my arm to fly back, beyond my range of motion and well outside my comfort zone. It was deep, bone-on-bone pain that brought tears to my eyes. I considered blowing off skiing the rest of the day. But when I got up and swung my arm around, whipping my ski pole through the air as a test, the left shoulder felt freer and moved with less pain. I think the sudden whiplash of it broke through some of the scar tissue in the shoulder and actually did me a lot of good. I iced the area

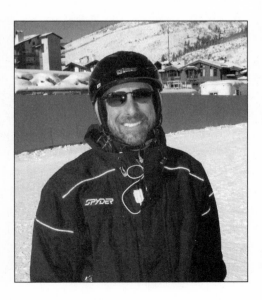

when I got home. I had considerable discomfort the next day, but my range of motion was hugely improved.

I could not shake the skiing accident from my mind. I'd retold the story to doctors, friends, and relatives, but still could not convince myself that it went down the way I recalled it. I knew my memory had been affected by the blackout and that the last seconds leading up to the fall were—and would remain—a mystery to me.

As an advanced skier, I am capable of negotiating bumps, "steeps," and tight, tree-lined trails. This was a simple wide-open slope, kid stuff. How could I be floating down the hill one minute and unconscious the next? Was it possible that I blacked out *before* the fall and that had precipitated the accident? If so, then how could I explain the intense impact that dislocated my left shoulder, cracked four ribs on my right side, and knocked me unconscious? Let's say that I did black out, that my body went limp and just collapsed onto the ski slope. Would this have produced the force to cause the damage that I suffered? Interestingly, I told the emergency room doctor at the Vail hospital that I had blacked out, but he did not order any tests. Would a CT scan or an MRI have shown evidence of a clot or some such thing that caused me to spontaneously lose consciousness?

I became obsessed with this, looking both ways on the ski slope like a kid crossing a busy street. I would fear skiing until I could get some closure. How dangerous would it be to pass out again at an even higher speed?

I drove to Snowmass a week later to join some friends from DC for a few days of skiing. I skied well the first day, but had to cut the second day short because of dizziness and a screaming headache. I didn't feel well enough to ski the next day, so I headed back to Boulder. I got another killer headache during the drive and was perplexed by the repeat performance. The altitude has done this to me before, but this felt different than a typical headache.

Chapter 3

THE EMERGENCY ROOM (APRIL 2, 2008 – DAY ONE)

B arbara helped me off the couch in the den and into the car. We pulled up to the emergency room at Boulder Community Hospital, and it took everything I had to get out of the car and stagger in. I felt disoriented and scared as I passed through the sliding electric doors and found my way to Admissions.

"I need to see a doctor now. I think I'm having a stroke."

Predictably, the woman behind the desk asked for my insurance card, and I fumbled with my wallet to produce it. But they asked only a few questions before they led me to the waiting room. Barb joined me there shortly, and a few minutes later I was escorted into an examining room and told—what else?—to wait. The doctor on duty came in and began asking questions, while the nurse took my vitals. I told him how I felt at the moment and recounted the events of the past few days.

While waiting for my MRI results, I had another headache and my arm went limp again. When the doctor told me that the imaging results looked normal and that I should be released shortly, I told him about the latest occurrence. He did not seem alarmed and suggested that I see my primary care physician soon.

I wanted to believe my problem was a pinched nerve and that the headaches, while different than my migraines, were associated. I waited some more, and was then told to get my "walking papers." To make things worse, I had two more TIAs while waiting in the ER.

The Second Diagnosis

I literally had my release papers in my hand when the phone rang at the nurse's desk in the ER. It was like the reverse version of the call that a death row inmate waits to receive from the governor, granting a stay of execution; it was the radiology department on the phone. A second radiologist had just reviewed my MRI.

The doctor said, "They found something on the MRI. You have to stay."

I looked questioningly at the doctor, confused and a bit scared.

"At least they found something conclusive, so you can be treated," he said. "You won't have to leave the hospital not knowing the cause of your problems and pain."

I can't say that I was all that relieved, but I nodded and feigned agreement as I walked slowly back to my examining room. They called Barb in from the waiting room, and then Dr. Alan Zacharias, the neurologist, and Dr. Jie Mao, an interventional radiologist. I was hooked up to an IV and given a blood thinner called heparin while we sat and waited for the explanation.

Dr. Zacharias spoke first. "You have a number of spots on your brain . . . blood clots. These clots represent the strokes that you've had over the past few days. You also have a dissection—a cut or a flap—in your right carotid artery. The flap narrowed the flow of blood through the artery, and your blood formed a clot on the flap. As this clot breaks off, the small pieces travel, along with blood flow, into your brain. These clots plug up small vessels in your brain, which cause strokes. We have to admit you."

"Now?" I asked. "I'd like to go home and get a change of clothes, get my life in order, and come back tomorrow."

"No, you have to be admitted now," said Dr. Zacharias. "We have to treat you *immediately.*"

Barb and I sat stunned, but alert and eager to hear what was next. I was a bit slow on the uptake, so Barb helped clarify things for me as the doctor described them in more detail.

"You have a couple of decisions to make, so let me explain your choices."

Barb nodded as Dr. Zacharias outlined the options.

"We can admit you to the ICU, start you on a blood thinner called Coumadin, and then watch you closely for a week. The goal is to thin your blood, both to prevent additional clots from forming and to allow your body to dissolve the clot that's formed on your carotid artery."

The doctor advocated this approach and believed it was the least invasive. The downsides: I could suffer one or more strokes during the week, which they would try to head off or negate, but a massive stroke was entirely possible.

Dr. Mao, the interventional radiologist, chimed in at this point to say that her mentor in Denver supported this approach as well.

If I went this route, I would be on Coumadin for a prolonged period, possibly a year or more. For a guy who had never been on a pharmaceutical before—other than an antibiotic once or twice—this scared me. When I asked them to expound, they described the known possible side effects of this drug: bruising and possible bleeding, high blood pressure, hemorrhage, and internal bleeding, to name a few.

Barb and I looked at each other and immediately rejected it.

"The other option?" I asked.

Dr. Mao started. "I understand that this is an accepted procedure, but I believe that the risk of stroke—and greater damage—is too great."

She pulled out a pad of paper and began sketching a diagram of the carotid artery, my tear or dissection, the subsequent "flap" that formed from the tear, the clot that formed on the flap, and, finally, the narrowed passage in the artery, which was estimated to be 60 percent blocked.

I won't get too scientific here, but this is what the procedure entailed: They would insert a catheter into the femoral artery in my groin and guide it up to the carotid artery in my neck. The carotid arteries are located on each side of the neck and are the main arteries supplying blood to the brain. They carry blood to the cerebral cortex, which is responsible for most of our day-to-day functioning.

Next, they would insert a collapsed stent into the line and send it up to the artery. The stent is a small wire mesh tube used to help keep the artery open. It is opened once it's in place. Besides opening the artery that was narrowed by the flap and clot, the stent would also press the clot against the artery wall to facilitate its absorption back into my system. Before placing the stent, they would send up an "umbrella," which is positioned above the location of the vessel damage to catch any clumps of clot that might be dislodged during the stent placement, hopefully catching them before they sprayed north into my brain. Dr. Mao told me that a rice-sized or even smaller piece of tissue could cause major paralysis or brain damage if it made it past the umbrella.

We asked how dangerous the stent procedure would be.

"All procedures carry risks," she replied. "In this case, we have to weigh the benefits and risks between the heparin and the stent, or the Coumadin and 'wait-and-see' method. You are having too many of these TIAs, and too frequently, despite full anticoagulation while you've been here in the ER. I believe the chance of your having a major stroke with the wait-and-see method is great, and that a stent placement now could prevent that." She added that after the procedure I would be on a less invasive blood thinner, such as Plavix—which still carries a number of side effects—for three to six months.

They both left the room for us to talk. Barb and I looked at each other, wide-eyed. She held my tingling hand as we shared a private and difficult moment. We tried to imagine me living with permanent paralysis or brain damage, and Barb having to nurse me. Given our distaste for and fear of prescription drugs, the uncertainty and time involved with the wait-and-see approach, my impatience, and the fact that Dr. Mao seemed so certain about her diagnosis and expectations, we decided to go with the stent and hope for the best. Dr. Mao gave us the necessary paperwork and told us that the procedure would be scheduled once the hospital confirmed it had the required stent. Until then, I would be on heparin.

I spent that night alone in the hospital ER, getting up regularly to visit the bathroom and stroll the halls, my IV in tow. Even in my fragile physical and mental state, I found the goings-on to be fascinating. I'd always had a fear of hospitals and had historically steered clear at all cost. Other than having our babies and visiting my father when he was fighting cancer, I'd kept my distance.

Nonetheless, I had grown to accept my little room over the last long hours and tried to make the best of it. It was like being in jail: I could watch, but I couldn't leave. Sleeping on the cold blue bed, with its icy steel and sliding sheets, did not come easily, and I found myself with lots of time on my hands. Reading was hard because I did not have my glasses.

During times of introspection—when visiting my father in the hospital and later in the care facility where he eventually died, or as I lay awake at night in my bed at home, or at times when I was feeling just a little *too* good, *too* fortunate—I had often wondered how I would cope with a major health problem should I ever find myself in that position. After much thought, and thanking God and my lucky stars, I had always decided that I'd be brave and positive. I'd think about the many unfortunate kids with cancer and other maladies and how brave they seemed to be. Daunting though it was, deep down I hoped and believed that I would cope and not lose my sense of humor.

Shortly after midnight I heard some shuffling and yelling in the hall outside my partially open door. I got up from the bed and peeked out. A male nurse and a couple of burly Boulder cops were dragging a long-haired guy in handcuffs and restraining chains into the room across from mine. The sight of cops, holsters, and what appeared to be a convict was a bit scary, but very exciting. The guy was restrained, so I didn't feel threatened, and it was just the diversion I needed to kill some time. The guy must have done something pretty bad to rank this kind of attention and supervision. Since he was face down, I could watch all I wanted with anonymity.

He was clearly becoming a problem for the ER staff that had to supervise him, so they injected him with a sedative, which angered him even more. He demanded to know why he was being sedated. The cops told him that he was out of control and they had no choice. Once they administered the sedative they closed his door, and that was the end of that drama.

Sleeping was tough that night. I may have drifted off, but I never made it to truly rejuvenating REM slumber. It appeared that the procedure was not going to happen that night, and I couldn't deal with it all. I rolled my IV rig out to the nurses' station and asked if they could give me a Valium or something to help me sleep.

"I'll have to check with the doctor on duty and get back to you."

Five minutes later, the nurse came in and injected liquid Valium into my IV. I can't say enough about the value of Valium in this form. I was asleep in a matter of seconds and did not wake until 6 AM. The ER was quiet when I woke, so I switched on the TV to pass time. It seemed like forever, but a nurse did eventually come to prep me for my procedure. Barb also came in, so they must have alerted her as well. We talked and hugged.

Dr. Mao stopped in to see how I was and assured me that I'd be going to the Operating Room soon. She said that the procedure would take forty minutes to an hour and that Barb should go to the waiting room; Dr. Mao would come see her after the procedure.

They rolled me to the operating room. Like most people, I had read about stroke and seen stroke victims depicted on TV and in movies, but none of it really registered with me on a deep, visceral level until that moment. Of all the anxieties that cloud our minds once we reach our fifties, I never imagined I might become a stroke victim. I ate well and exercised, I probably had clean, plaque-free arteries, and I didn't have a family history of strokes. I had retired from a stressful vocation seven years before and lived a very peaceful life in the foothills of Colorado.

Chapter 4

LIFE AS I KNEW IT "PRE-STROKE"

I love tennis and play three times a week. Because of my passion for the game, I earned my teaching certification at fifty-two years of age. I dance, hike, bike, and ski. I started rollerblading at the age of forty, and have since bladed the streets of New York City, San Diego, Los Angeles, and London. I also love the ocean, have bodysurfed since I was a kid, and have taught both of my sons, who are very good athletes. My wife, Barbara, dances four times a week and trained in Pilates, which she also taught. In short, as a family we are all physically active.

In 1986, after Barbara and I had built, operated, and sold a successful dance and active-wear clothing store in Ann Arbor, Michigan, we moved our family back to my hometown of Bethesda, Maryland, just outside Washington, DC. We sold the clothing store so I could return to our family's third-generation dry cleaning business. I worked the business until 1994 and then bought my father's flagship store, the "crown jewel." We spent—God help me—fifteen years running the business. In 2001 I sold the cleaners and began writing books on clothing care and consulted with dry cleaners and consumers around the country.

I was one of those "hands-on" owners, creative and engaged. I woke every day with the energy to lead the world. I descended on the cleaners like a fire-breathing dragon ready to slay the enemy—though I wasn't always sure who the enemy was. Some days it was me, some days the customer, and some days it was the employees. I worked with a passion and could not be derailed.

I went into the dry cleaning business to use my creativity and to make money, and found it to be the ultimate outlet for a type A personality like myself. I was a natural-born entrepreneur and had owned three businesses before getting into the dry cleaning world. I believed that the dry cleaners was a place to *work*, plain and simple, and could never cozy up to the idea of a lax work environment. Some of my employees respected my passion and focus, but it scared most of them. I had no time for small talk, unless it had the potential to instruct, refine, or grow the business.

My home life suffered because of the long hours, and I missed both my sons' after-school games. Barb had her hands full, but she understood what it took to run our crazy enterprise. This doesn't mean that she enjoyed having to raise the kids alone or that I didn't feel guilty, but we did earn the money to put both our boys through private school, which was a priority for us.

By age forty-three, I was feeling disillusioned and angry with myself for missing so much of my children's growth. Abandoning my eighty-hour weeks, I started leaving work each day at three to catch their games, and I stopped working Saturdays completely. From that point on, I attended almost every basketball and soccer game they played. This lifestyle change probably saved me from a full-blown stroke. At the same time, I began working on my exit strategy from the dry cleaning business. I'd had it with the long hours, the broken machinery, the labor issues, and the growing restrictions from the EPA and OSHA.

At forty-six, with much luck and excellent timing, I sold the business and entered semi-retirement. Retirement at forty-six—I had to pinch myself. After twenty-five years of work, with only a week off each year, I was in uncharted territory. I reported for "work" every day for the next three months as part of my agreement with the new owner, but I had no responsibility to speak of. The time flew by, and before I knew it I was on my own.

For the next six months I played tennis, rollerbladed, and ice-skated. I spent lots of time with Barb and my sons. I rolled out of bed early, but instead of heading to work at the cleaners, I went to the computer and wrote. I had started my first book while running the business, but was so zapped of energy when I got home each night that I had nothing left in my creative tank. After acclimating to life at home, I began "sleeping in" till six or seven, writing until noon or so, and then doing something physical. I picked up Ben after school, went to his and Bryan's games, and slowly became semi-retired.

I could not have been happier, but my body was hurting from constant exercise and sport. I had no idea that semi-retirement could be so hard! I had trouble finding enough guys my age to play with, as the other retired men I met were considerably older. Most people my age were busy building careers and living the lives of workaholics, just as I had done.

Barb and I talked about spending more time together: riding bikes and taking walks, maybe even playing a bit of tennis. We did some of this, but she, too, had her agenda and was very busy with Pilates and running errands for the house. Barb liked her "alone" time at home while the kids were at school, and I was cramping her style by always being underfoot. She grew tired of me being home every day and thought that it was time for me to start doing something constructive.

My semi-retirement had drastically altered Barb's day-to-day routine—one that she had maintained for most of the years that I worked and the boys were in school. I knew little of this life of hers. She started leaving the house and staying away for most of the day. She dropped subtle hints, such as leaving newspaper articles on my desk about other "retirees" and how their spouses were going nuts having their husbands at home. In Japan, for example, women were actually becoming ill from the presence of their retired husbands. They had to cook, cater, and wait on them hand and foot. The Japanese women developed ulcers and other stress-related diseases, and the men were oblivious. This was not our problem, but I got the drift.

I continued to write every morning, often till mid-afternoon, and sometimes late into the night. The solitary time was good for me after so many years of stimulation. I locked myself up in our home office and wrote like a demon for eighteen months until I had finished *The Ultimate Guide to Shopping & Caring for Clothing,* one of the most intriguing and thorough books on clothing care ever published (if I do say so myself), and the first of its kind.

The clothing-care book became my passport into the world of the consumer, granting me access to radio, newspaper, and television interviews. I learned that writing a book could make you an expert in the eyes of the media. I became *The Clothing Doctor®* to millions of consumers and thousands of dry cleaners. Brands such as Frigidaire, Tide, OxiClean, Clorox, and Whirlpool hired me and contributed to projects to help educate consumers.

During those first years, and after publishing my first book, I appeared as a guest on *The View* with Barbara Walters and on *Good Day New York,* and was a frequent contributor to clothing-care segments on NBC, CBS, and CNN. I wrote and hosted a national radio show called "The Clothing Doctor" on WOR in New York City, and commuted weekends from Bethesda to New York for almost a year. I built a second career around The Clothing Doctor and have continued writing books and making instructional videos for dry cleaners and consumers.

Chapter 5

SURGERY DAY—THE ACTUAL PROCEDURE (APRIL 3, 2008)

I was rolled into the OR and transferred to the operating table. Now I felt vulnerable, though still secure in my decision to have the stent procedure. They lifted my hospital gown and told me that they would have to shave my groin area to insert the catheter into the femoral artery. At this point, after almost twenty-four hours in the grip of hospital life, I had very few inhibitions. I was given a few shots to numb the area and off they went.

Dr. Mao reviewed the procedure with me and then signaled her team to put me under twilight anesthesia. They wanted me "awake" during the operation so I could tell them how I was doing, and if I had feeling in my limbs. I felt the catheter line going up my body. I don't know how much time passed, but they were all talking quietly, while watching the screen during the insertion of the stent.

At some point the chatting turned louder and more clipped, and the OR team seemed to be moving more furiously. They asked how I was doing, and I whispered, "Fine." All of a sudden, I started feeling strange. Dr. Mao asked whether I could move my left hand and my fingers . . . and if I had feeling in my feet and elsewhere in my body. I nodded in the affirmative, but I was not feeling right. I spoke directly to her, but could not identify with the voice coming from my mouth.

"My left hand and arm are rippling," I said. "They feel wet and cold, like water running through my skin."

I couldn't see if my arm was moving or shaking, but it was the strangest sensation I'd ever experienced. I couldn't directly identify with what was happening around me, but there was commotion amongst the team. They asked again if I could feel my hands and feet, and could I move them, which I did. They asked me to push my foot against the nurse's hand at the end of the table, which I did. That's about all I remember.

The Recovery Room

I awoke in the recovery room with the most intense and painful headache I've ever had. It was worse than the headaches I had during my TIAs and worse than the vise grip I used to feel during my most severe migraines. Dr. Mao's face swam before me. I was out of it, but able to explain to her how I felt, and they quickly gave me something for the pain. As the pain subsided, she began to explain what had occurred during surgery. She was, first of all, relieved to hear that I could speak and did not have any facial contortions or speech impediments— something I had not even considered amongst my physiological issues.

"The procedure was a success and the stent is in place," she continued. "All of your arteries were very clean, with no plaque or build-up, which is a great thing. But because the artery was so clean, it treated the stent like an invader and went into extreme spasm when the stent was inserted in the carotid artery. If there had been some plaque to coat the artery, it would not have reacted so violently."

In short, I'd had another stroke during the surgery, one which would later turn out to have caused greater and longer-lasting damage than my earlier TIAs. The team had worked fast and furiously to minimize the danger and damage by injecting me with Reopro, an anti-platelet agent, more heparin, and nitroglycerin for spasm. It was during this time that they started asking me questions and I felt that bizarre ripple through my arm. A few days later Dr. Mao told me how nervous she'd been during the procedure when the spasm occurred.

"I was shitting bricks!"

Even in my beleaguered state, I had a good laugh.

Chapter 6

ASSESSING THE DAMAGE

In the face of shock and loss, a strange calm had washed over me. I'd come out of surgery in one piece—a broken piece, true, but I was alive. As I gazed around it began to sink in. I was in the Intensive Care Unit, and I had suffered a stroke. Yesterday I'd been out in the world with full use of my brain and body, and today I was—well, I wasn't exactly sure what I now was. But of one thing I was certain: My life had changed.

That day I had my first visit from James, a physical therapist. They had wasted no time on this step, and I was glad. James, a buff, soft-spoken guy in his thirties, had brought all kinds of devices in his bag of tricks. He wanted to get a baseline reading to establish my physical condition directly after surgery. James began by testing my right side, which was a little weak, but okay. My left side was another story. I had a bag of almonds on the tray near me. James dumped a few onto the surface of the tray.

"Can you pick up an almond with your left hand?" he asked.

I was still woozy from the influence of Percocet every few hours, but I gave a confident little laugh, thinking, *Why don't you ask me to do something difficult?* As it turned out, this task wasn't just difficult, it was impossible. I could position my hand to hover over the almond, but could not zero in to close my fingers around it, much less actually pinch it. My hand had suffered severe paralysis. I looked at James in confusion and he gently asked me to keep trying, but to take my time. I simply could not do it, no matter how persistently I willed my limb to do my bidding.

James smiled and told me, "Pay it no mind; we'll work on it." Next, he pulled out a large, wide fork and spoon, with padded rubber handles for easier grip and manipulation. My father had used a set of these when he was in the hospital suffering from neuropathy during his cancer chemotherapy.

I tried holding the spoon, but could not grip it, even with the wide handle. James adjusted my hand position, but I still could not rotate my hand to hold it with the spoon part up. If I'd had soup in the spoon it would have spilled. In order to do this, and many other things, I would later learn to pronate my hand (rotate the hand so that the palm faced down), or supinate my hand (rotate the hand so that the palm faced up, like a soup bowl). This would prove to be a very challenging part of my recovery, on many levels.

James gave me a small Tupperware container of hot pink Silly Putty-like goop, which they call Thera-Putty, to squeeze and shape. This, along with the fat flatware, was geared to help me relearn the basics as I worked to articulate my finger movements.

My last therapy homework of the day was a finger exercise in which I had to touch my thumb to my forefinger, then my middle, ring, and finally, my pinky finger. This, I learned, was typical protocol for every stroke victim with paralysis. Months later I would see other stroke survivors doing this every day as a matter of practice and discipline, like someone fidgeting with worry beads. But for now, I could not get my left thumb to touch even one finger.

I'd had no idea how hobbled I was until this first session, but James radiated confidence that I would succeed. He encouraged me to remain hopeful and patient. I had my work and goals cut out for me, and I would have plenty of time to practice between my therapy sessions and the constant visits from the ICU nurses taking my vitals.

Barb came to visit and gave me an update on life outside the hospital walls, as she tried to carry on without me for a bit. She'd been emailing updates to my mother and siblings, and to her family. Both our sons were frightened and anxious, and didn't really know how to react, as they'd never seen either of their parents in the hospital or in such a precarious and vulnerable condition. They still considered us too young for such madness. Ben had a jump start on my mortality because he had nursed me through my ski accident at Vail.

I'd been thinking about the time Barb spent in the waiting room during the operation, so I asked her to tell me about it. She said it was one of the most stressful and traumatic experiences of her life. Dr. Mao had told her that the procedure would take less than an hour, if all went well. She waited almost two hours, terrified as each minute ticked by that something had gone terribly wrong.

I felt terrible for Barb. I knew her worst times are usually in the middle of the night, when she wakes from a bizarre dream and can't get back to sleep. Her mind races through issues that would be manageable during the day, but seem so intense and blown out of proportion in the dark. And that's when I'm home, next to her in bed! For her to sleep alone, with me in the ICU, would be even darker for her. I did my best to comfort her and reassure her that I would recover.

Barb was still in the room when Jennifer, another physical therapist, walked in. As it turned out, she and Barb knew each other from yoga class. They laughed about the coincidence and chatted for a few minutes. This is one of the most amazing things about the small-town Boulder vibe. If I'd been in the hospital back in DC, there would be almost no chance that we'd know the therapist.

Jennifer, a cheerful blond of about thirty-five, had come to assess my vision and cognitive ability. She started with a simple reading chart, a mix of words and images. She asked me to read a few lines of text. Barb pulled my reading glasses from her bag, and I started. I could recognize the letters, but they were all bunched together and cramped. As I strained to read aloud, I thought I did well, considering. As it turned out, I missed the first word on every line. The test was also very fatiguing.

Next Jennifer gave me some very simple line drawings of a house, much like the pictures little kids draw. She asked me to copy what I saw, line for line. I had a very hard time understanding or perceiving what I saw. I copied it as well as I could with my right hand and gave it back. I had completely missed the left part of the house, much like I had missed the first word of each sentence.

Jennifer explained that I had what they call a "left field cut." This meant that my vision, mostly on the left, was considerably diminished and impaired. I might be seeing objects with both eyes, but the left side was not registering visual information. In a soothing tone, Jennifer explained that it was a common condition with stroke survivors and that it should get better in time, with therapy and practice.

"Let's try some verbal tests, so you don't have to read or draw," she suggested.

She read off a string of five items and asked me to repeat them in the same exact order. She did the same with a string of numbers. I was frustrated and confused because I could not do either of them. Then she read a brief "situation," much like the story problems from the SATs, but easier. She began, "Jane had two dollars for a snack. She got a muffin for eight-five cents and a juice for fifty cents. She gave the cashier the money. How much change did she get back? Take your time and give me the answer when you can."

I thought about it and thought about it, trying to do the math in my head. I'd handled this exact kind of exchange thousands of times before without trouble, but this time I just couldn't follow the process.

The therapy session was a humbling and depressing experience. It would take time and a lot of work—both physical and mental—to get me feeling normal again. I was starting to imagine myself being stuck in rehab for months, even years, and it scared me.

Jennifer left me some pictures to copy and some reading to do when I felt up to it. She bid us goodbye and said we'd do it all again the next day.

Barb hung out for a bit and consoled me. I was overwhelmed and exhausted. I kept the drawings, the bag of almonds, and the Thera-Putty near the bed and resolved to practice when I had the energy.

Chapter 7

ICU—DAY TWO

I had not really walked since the procedure, but I had to get to the toilet in my room, so it was time to try. I couldn't lift myself out of bed, even with one good hand, so I got help from one of the many nurses. Feeling a bit like a boat in the surf, I hobbled over to the toilet in the corner of the room and sat down. Muscle loss and atrophy happen fast when you're completely bedridden, so it was painful to move—but it felt right. And it was liberating not having to use a bedpan again.

I used the opportunity to take a short stroll around the ICU. Seeing a bunch of sick people hooked up to dripping tubes and beeping monitors was hardly a stroll on the beach, but the freedom that came with walking around on my own was almost as sweet. I was hunched over and stiff, like someone with a bad flu, gingerly holding a blanket around my shoulders with my good hand as I did two loops around the ICU desk. I noticed a computer on the counter and asked if it would be okay to try using it. I was anxious to see if I could use the mouse and type a few words into the Google bar. To my dismay, I found that I could not.

One of my nurses, seeing that I was mobile, suggested that we take a short walk outside. I was shocked to find that this was an option and told her yes — anything to get some fresh air and to commune with nature. Outdoors it was sunny and breezy, a beautiful spring day. I hadn't seen the sun or blue skies since my ride to the emergency room—eons ago, it seemed.

There I stood, in my hospital garb, the open slit in the back flapping in the wind, a white knitted blanket over my shoulders like a granny's shawl, taking wobbly baby steps. My hair, which I am usually self-conscious about, had gone unwashed and uncombed for three days. This was not The Clothing Doctor's finest fashion statement—but I didn't give a shit! It still amazes me how uninhibited we become when we're in the hospital.

Back from my short adventure, energized with fresh air and the sight of "free" people walking around outside the ER, I got back into bed and spaced out a bit. I must have been getting a little better because I thought about food for the first time. When Barb called to see how I was feeling, I asked her to bring me something tasty to eat.

Thirty minutes later she had not arrived, but my hospital lunch did. Today's feast was a Sloppy Joe sandwich, with what looked like gravy-soaked brisket. I picked up my fat fork to sample the pieces that had fallen out of the bun. I was famished, so I cheated and used my right hand to eat. Not bad— almost tasty, even. Then I picked up the sandwich with both hands, using my left hand to support the bun, and devoured the first few bites.

Resting for a moment, I looked down to find my left hand nestled in the potatoes and gravy. I hadn't even felt it. I laughed at the absurdity of it all. It's been said that old people revert to childhood as they age, an interesting role reversal, with their children taking care of them. Well, there's nothing like a stay in the ICU to make you feel as useless as a newborn baby. I finished eating and was glad to be through with it.

I still felt energized, so I began work on my therapy exercises. I started with the almonds, my greatest nemesis. I laid a few almonds on the bed tray and committed myself to beating this thing. I was primed for a championship bout: Three almonds versus me. I tried like the devil to position my left hand with the palm down, hovering over an almond like one of those arcade claws in a glass case that swoops down to grab a stuffed animal or some knickknack. It would look like a sure thing until the toy slowly slipped out of the grasp of the claw and back into the collection of trinkets.

I took a deep breath. All I had to do was drop my hand onto the almond, squeeze my thumb and forefinger together, and pinch it. I willed myself down to the almond and, like a super-slow-motion replay on ESPN, I forced myself to grasp the waiting nut. It took almost a full minute, but I got it in my grip and lifted it. Beaming, I looked around to share my accomplishment with someone, but I was the only one in sight—and quite honestly, the only one who mattered.

This was a meaningful step and a valuable lesson. Except for the time I spent with physical therapists, most of my accomplishments would be solitary endeavors, just for me: an ultimate challenge, no frills, no fanfare, and no "attaboys" from Mom or Dad. This was my cross to bear and my mountain to climb.

I grasped the almond for a few seconds and then excitedly dropped it onto the tray to try another one, as quickly as possible. I picked up the second almond in fifteen seconds!

I learned another valuable lesson, one that would buoy and strengthen my resolve: Most of the fundamentals that we take for granted, such as brushing our teeth, tying our shoes, drinking from a glass, washing dishes, and zipping our pants, do not come back to stroke survivors simply because we once knew how to do them. We have to relearn them. We no longer have the original "pathways" in our brain to perform these tasks, so we have to forge new ones. In this case, I had created a new neural pathway to squeeze my fingers together to pick up the almond. But once I did, it became a part of my new world, making the next attempt that much easier. This was a monumental discovery.

I dropped that second almond and began picking up another and another. I was always up for a challenge, whether it was hitting a tennis ball, doing a flip off a diving board for the first time, or learning to rollerblade at forty. As someone who derives joy from learning new skills, I was not easily dissuaded or intimidated.

By the time "Gentle James," my therapist, returned the next day, I could pick up an almond almost at will. Excited for me, he grinned and gave me those "attaboys." But he also pointed out that I was cheating; I had been contorting my hand and arm to pick up the almond sideways, using the wrong body mechanics. I would never be able to hold a glass of water or carry a plate like this without spilling.

I was a bit discouraged and affronted by the rain on my parade after all my work. Hadn't I accomplished something monumental? Well yes, I had. But I would also have to learn to appreciate correction in the face of accomplishment, accept constructive criticism, and get over it.

We spent about twenty minutes on hand position, handling the fork and spoon, squeezing putty, and touching my thumb to each finger. I used my right hand to help touch my left thumb to the fingers, but James assured me that this was okay for now. We were retraining my brain. He encouraged me, and told me again that I was doing very well. Then he told me that this would be our last session together, as he was going camping with his kids for a week. He smiled his gentle smile at my forlorn expression and said that in two weeks time I'd be onto many other endeavors in an outpatient program at Boulder Rehabilitation. He wished me luck and said that he knew I would be fine. I thanked him and told him to have a great time with his kids. I'd already grown to deeply appreciate the commitment and focus of my various therapists.

When Barb picked up my meal, she'd seen our friends Mamie and Barry sitting outside. After hearing about my stroke, they decided to come for a visit. I hadn't known that I could have visitors other than family in the ICU, so it was a pleasant surprise seeing the two of them come in. I got a kiss from Mamie, as always. Barry gave me a high-five and presented me with a pair of big red boxing gloves.

He said, "You're a fighter! You should have these!"

I was a fighter. I still looked like hell, was miles from feeling normal, and I couldn't handle the gloves; but I felt deeply touched and entertained by the sentiment and the gift. I thanked him and felt his smile.

I was feeling pretty worn out, so after a little while Mamie and Barry said their goodbyes. It was sweet to see friends from beyond the hospital walls, and I was thrilled and truly moved that they'd taken the time to come. Now, though, I needed to rest.

That afternoon, a nurse came in to remove the catheter line in my femoral artery. I'd been sedated when they inserted it in the operating room, so all I remembered was the nurse shaving the area and feeling a little pull inside my skin. The removal proved to be a bit more interesting as they pulled the three-foot line from my body. This was a huge event, because it was the last tie I had to the ICU. Tomorrow I'd be moving into the rehab wing at the hospital.

Chapter 8

THE REHAB WING

I was anxious to get out of the ICU for two reasons. First, I wanted a room with a shower and a private bathroom, instead of a toilet in plain sight. Second, moving out of the ICU would signify my improved condition. I said goodbye to the nurses on the night shift and thanked them for their care and attention. I felt amazed by how close I'd grown to these people. They were my lifelines, and they made a crucial difference to me.

I was wheeled up to rehab and deposited into my own room. I felt relieved just to be there. It had been a long three days, and I had officially survived! In two more days I might be discharged, if everything went well. Despite my exhaustion, I longed to take my first shower. There were two nurses on the night shift in my section. The pretty younger nurse set up my room, asked if I needed any food or a video, took my vitals of course, and showed me the call button in case I needed something during the night. An older nurse came in to help supervise my shower.

Moving slowly, and still very shaky on my own two feet, I started to get out of my smock. My nurse pointed out the shampoo and soap, and then offered to help me shower. As much as I wanted to do this for myself, I couldn't. The nurse helped me out of the hospital garb and into the shower stall. The orange disinfectant they used to shave my groin was still there, a reminder of that scary and stressful period as they prepped me for the stent procedure. I held onto the support bar with my right hand and waved her off. On her way out, she left me a pair of pajamas—actual tops and bottoms, with no slits or open areas. I was moving on up!

The hot water felt delicious and enveloping, and the privacy was almost like life on the outside. I used my good hand to pour the shampoo into the palm of my bad hand. Unable to supinate—to keep my left palm open and level to hold the shampoo—it flowed right off the surface, like cooking oil from a frying pan with no sides, and onto the shower floor. I laughed and tried a different tack. I laid the shampoo bottle on its side with the spout hanging off the edge of the seat in the shower stall, put my right hand under the spout, and pushed down on the bottle with my left hand. With a jerky motion, I got the shampoo onto my head and moved it around with my right hand until it began to lather. Success! This was real life, on my own. I soaped up, tried to play with myself just to see if it still worked (it did), and then rinsed off. I finished the shower feeling triumphant.

My left hand and arm were really quite useless. My shoulder was frozen from the dislocation and nerve damage from the stroke, and my arm just hung there, numb and lifeless. I had been rehabbing my left shoulder when I got the stroke, but it still had a limited range of motion. When the stroke hit the nerves on the left side, it negated any rehab work I'd done on the shoulder. Drying off was a challenge—as everything would prove to be with one lame wing—and it took five minutes to get into the pajamas they gave me. I didn't bother brushing my hair, but I emerged from the bathroom feeling like a new man.

Up till then, I hadn't had much time or energy to reflect on my condition and what it would mean to me in the long term. I knew having a stroke would undoubtedly change my life in many ways. There would be life lessons and hard times, as I would endure painful and challenging rehabilitation. But these considerations were still abstract. The few minutes I spent alone in the bathroom now opened my sedated eyes and foggy brain to just a few of these issues.

Hospitals are not the place to get quality rest and undisturbed sleep. That night they woke me at least three times for vitals and such. Even in the privacy of my own room, I could hear activity in the hall all night long. I woke around 5:30 AM and lay in silence for an hour, until the morning nurse came in. The rehab wing was bustling, and I could see that the sun was shining outside my window.

Later that morning a nurse came in to listen to my chest and lungs. She observed some congestion, and as there is danger of pneumonia for bedridden people, she brought me a spirometer—a plastic contraption for measuring lung capacity. I'd have to breathe in as deeply as I could and then exhale for as long as I could, then read the marks on the side to get the measurement. I was told to do this every twenty-five minutes for the next day or so. She also had some concern about blood flow to my legs, given the time I'd been in bed. She hooked me up to some vibrating boots to stimulate blood flow. I must have been better the next morning, because they removed the boots and took back the spirometer.

Life in the Rehabilitation Wing

I had a visit from a nutritionist on my first morning in rehab. She wanted to discuss my meals while in the hospital, and what I should eat when I got out. The hospital actually offered a menu for meals, which made me laugh. Did the choices really mean anything? I might have scarfed down the Sloppy Joe, but wasn't it all the same tasteless dreck? I decided on pancakes, a slice of bacon, some orange juice, and a cup of decaf.

What I really want to know is when hospitals will start serving healthy foods—foods that actually contain vitamins and minerals, and that won't clog your arteries and land you back in the hospital! Many months later I saw this cartoon in *Parade* magazine and I had to include it in this book. I wrote Gary

McCoy for permission to reprint it and he gladly approved. (His dad had suffered a stroke weeks earlier and complained about the same thing!)

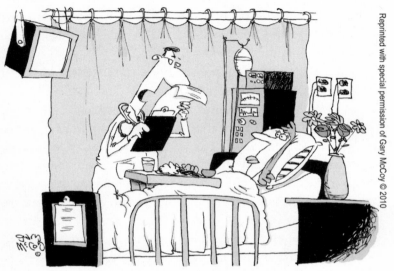

"If you ever hope to improve your health, you've got to stop eating hospital food."

Filled and fueled with soggy pancakes and cold, fatty bacon, I got out of bed to take a slow walk around the rehab wing. I ventured into the hall. Besides the nurses and the other basic reminders that this was a hospital, the place seemed more like a hotel. The floors were carpeted, there was wallpaper, and it smelled less like a hospital than it had in the ICU.

I grabbed a wheelchair to use as a walker as I struggled up a gently angled ramp. It was almost as challenging as hiking. I followed the hallway that led to some built-in shelves with books, magazines, and videos. To the left was a rehab room with steps, ramps, climbing apparatus, fitness balls, and other cool stuff. I surveyed the video shelf. As hard as it was to read the titles, I chose a few for that night, which I carried in my right hand.

On the way back to my room, I saw a laminated poster on the wall. It was obviously a diagram of the brain; I recognized that much. I scanned the two-line title at the top, which seemed to read *he rain*. I knew that was wrong and looked again to realize that it said, "The Brain." I cracked up; it seemed to me the funniest, most poignant mishap that I was unable to read a simple phrase like "The Brain" because of my own brain! I knew that because of my left vision cut I was having trouble reading the letters furthest to the left. I wanted to study the poster to learn more about the brain and my stroke. I reread the title and felt a little better when I actually saw the "B" in "Brain" this time.

Later, a very attractive woman came in and introduced herself as Leslie, my rehab therapy person for the next day or so. She would also be the person to decide whether I would be moved to a formal inpatient rehab floor or be scheduled for outpatient rehab once I was discharged. She checked out my hand and arm responses, then announced that we'd be going to the rehab room, the one I'd seen before with all the equipment.

Leslie walked with me to the workout room, offering help, which I graciously declined. Once in the room, I was excited to be doing something physical, as limited as it may have been. We started on the ramp, which felt like a steep cliff. I held the handrail and slowly moved up and down a few times, each step a little more surefooted than the last, but far from normal.

I noticed a basketful of balls, from tennis balls to various small bouncing balls, as well as a few large medicine balls on the floor along the edge of the room. Leslie asked me to toss and then catch a tennis ball with my right hand. I figured it would be a breeze, since it was my dominant hand and the relatively unaffected side of my body. I was terrible, missing the catch almost every time. The stroke had "stroked" my whole body, not just my left arm, hand, shoulder, and vision and brain functions.

Next, Leslie tossed me a lightweight medicine ball the size of a basketball, which I tried to catch with both hands. After a lifetime of ball games, I was stunned when it dropped out of both hands, repeatedly. I could not catch even a small ball in my left hand. We went through a series of hand-eye coordination exercises, my strong suit from tennis, golf, and juggling. She gently reassured me that I had done well for the first time and that it would get better and better with practice; something I would hear often in the coming months.

Relearning these fundamentals was a bizarre process. Pre-stroke, I could do all of these things with ease and confidence. Now it felt like I was five years old again, learning the basics for the first time. Even if I had the physical prowess to accomplish the task, it seemed I had neither the functional memory nor the muscle memory for these basic actions. I returned to my bed feeling more alive, but a bit depressed.

Barb and I had spoken earlier about her bringing dinner. My appetite had returned fully, and I was craving a grilled burger and hand-cut fries from one of my favorite restaurants in Boulder.

I was certainly feeling better. With some concerns and guarded expectations, I'd be ready in a day or two to leave the hospital and fend for myself at home. To accomplish this, I'd need one more CT angiogram to assess the condition of the stent placement. I was told that the doc would check my charts, and if all looked favorable, he would schedule the CT scan for the next day.

I was in a deep sleep that night, zonked out on two Percocets, when I felt something foreign touch my body that completely freaked me out. I woke instantly, roused from a drug-induced space in another world. My numb dead hand had touched my face for just a moment. It was the weirdest sensation. Since the hand was numb, it felt totally alien on my face, like it was someone else who was touching me. I literally jumped up in a cold sweat, my heart pounding like a sledge-hammer. After realizing what had happened, I tucked my arm by my side and went back to sleep.

My Last Day in the Hospital

I woke early, feeling decent, even after the strange night of sleep. I ate breakfast, took a walk around the rehab floor, and then settled back in to hopefully hear from Dr. Zacharias.

In the meantime, I had another visitor, an old friend from childhood who was in town visiting his daughters at the University of Colorado. Marc and I had skied together in Snowmass my last time out, and he'd just spent a few days at Beaver Creek and Vail.

I told him about the stroke and my theory about sustaining the damage to my carotid artery from the ski accident. I now believed that the impact from the hit-and-run had caused the dissection to the carotid artery and the subsequent "flap" that caused the growth of the blood clot. Marc said that he'd almost gotten nailed on the slope that week. A guy who was really moving down the hill took a jump and whizzed right past him, just missing his head. He completely understood how I could get hit.

I showed him my newfound ability to pick up an almond with my left hand, and we talked about his girls and shot the shit for a while. It was great of him to visit and hang out—a terrific diversion, helping me kill some nervous time.

The nurse came in to confirm my CT scan for three o'clock. I was just plain nervous and overwhelmed by all of this. I was afraid that the tests might show another dissection or clot. I felt vulnerable and out of my element. Reading was impossible because of my vision, so I watched TV to take my mind off the impending CT scan. Finally a nurse wheeled me down to radiology; the tests were done quickly, and I was wheeled back to my room. Now I just had to wait. If we got good news, I'd be out of the hospital today. Bad news . . . I couldn't fathom bad news, but the anxiety was worse than waiting for the initial results in the ER.

Sitting up on the side of my bed, I reflected on my five-day stay in the hospital. It already felt like a month. I couldn't wait to get home, to sleep in my own bed, to eat real food when I wanted, and to get the hell off the Percocet. I was sure that much of my depression and physical lethargy was a result of the painkillers I was taking every day and night.

Dr. Zacharias came in that afternoon with the results. "Everything looks good, and you can go home today."

I instantly relaxed. The conversation turned to my life outside the hospital. The doctor explained that I would be on Plavix, a blood thinner, for three to six months. I shouldn't rush back into activities, but I shouldn't be afraid, either. I would start physical therapy and occupational therapy on an outpatient basis as soon as I was ready, though I was forbidden to drive for the time being. Dr. Zacharias warned me to be patient on many levels, as recovery from stroke is not measured in weeks, but in months and possibly years.

I didn't argue. He did, however, try to impress upon me a very important point: I was technically fine. I had no obstructions, no plaque, and no evidence of clots. I should return to my daily schedule of work and exercise as soon as I was physically and mentally able. Knowing that I'm a physical guy, he assured me that I should not be concerned or fearful about hiking, biking, or tennis. I would meet with him in one month, and then have a follow-up CT scan in three months.

I started gathering my few possessions, which consisted mostly of the physical therapy toys I'd been given. I couldn't do much with one hand, and my shoulder was still frozen, but I was very relieved to be going home.

Chapter 9

HOME AT LAST

Iwalked into our beautiful home in time to see the place basking in the rosy light of the setting sun, welcoming and warm. As I moved slowly to my sofa in the den, I looked at my guitar, wondering if I dared take a strum. I also had a computer downstairs in the office, with no less than five hundred unanswered or undeleted emails. I felt the first pang of responsibility. My hospital stay may have been freaky, scary, and otherworldly, with way too many decisions to make about my health and future, but I'd had no real responsibilities; everything was done *for* me. Home represented work and challenge, on many levels.

I stood in front of my little work desk in the kitchen next to the stove and was immediately reminded that I'd gone almost a full week without taking my vitamins. I laid out my prescription slip for Plavix on the countertop, which Barb would fill for me the next day. My notepad, which usually contained a few messages from Barb, was blank except for a few unfinished chores that I would have crossed off, had I been home the previous week. Just the thought of doing a chore in my condition weighed on me heavily.

I shrugged off my unbuttoned denim shirt to realize that the IV port was still in my right arm. In the excitement around my leaving the hospital, the nurse must have forgotten to remove it. I started laughing, knowing Barb is very squeamish about this sort of thing. Noticing the IV, she freaked out and flatly refused to help remove it, stating succinctly that I'd have to go back to the hospital to have it taken out.

I said, "We can remove this at home, but you will have to do it!"

She wasn't happy, but I insisted that there was no way I was going back to the hospital anytime soon. She called the rehab wing and spoke to the nurse who had supervised my discharge. The nurse apologized for overlooking the IV and kindly explained how to remove the port and the needle. I used to watch medical procedures on PBS, and I also watched the birth of our boys, so I considered this little procedure doable. We pulled out the scissors and carefully cut off the gauze and tape. Then, pushing the tube and needle flat to my skin, we gingerly slid out the needle. Barb shook and squirmed, adorable as always.

Now I was really home, and it was time to settle in. I quickly realized that there was very little I could do to pass the time: reading was out, as I couldn't focus on the written word and I couldn't really understand what I was reading. I usually did the dishes since Barb cooked, but that was out because I couldn't hold a dish or a glass. Barb told me to just sit on the couch and relax, and that she would make dinner while I watched some TV. I obliged.

My guitar stood on its stand in the corner, looking very inviting, but playing anything on it was inconceivable. On any given day before the stroke I would have played for thirty minutes or so, practicing scales and songs I'd been working on. Now I picked up the guitar with trepidation and began to strum with my right hand, which was not 100 percent, but was certainly more responsive and capable than the limb on the left that normally had the hard job of forming the notes and chords.

I placed my left hand over the strings on the fret board and naturally gravitated to the D-chord—a three-finger chord I had learned at nine years old and could play in my sleep. I could not play even a single note, much less form a chord. For all of the non-guitar-players reading this, playing a D-chord is as fundamental as holding a fork. I tried a different approach, pressing one finger on one note on one string. My limp and completely spastic forefinger could not hold a single note. After a lifetime of playing guitar, I was speechless. I put the guitar back on its stand and judiciously left it for another day.

I ambled tentatively down the stairs that led to my office, holding onto the rail for support. I sat in my small but enveloping office with the amazing view of the foothills and reservoir. The computer screen stared me in the face. I struggled to hit a few numbers and letters on the keyboard to pull up my inbox and began to survey my email from the past week. Using my right hand, I moved the mouse to scroll up and down. I saw a huge number of messages and attempted to read a few, as they were just a few lines each. But between the size of the type and the pulsating electronic letters, it was like reading gibberish. I stared at the screen for minutes on end, unable to comprehend even one message. I gave it up and went back to the den, completely overwhelmed.

I ate some dinner, watched a movie with half my attention, and then showered. Barb came in with me to help with the soap and the shampoo. It felt good to get the hospital smell off me.

I also found out that my loins were alive and wanting, but I did not have the energy to partake. The discovery was comforting, though.

I dried off, again with Barb's help, and went up to bed. As snug and welcoming as my bed and clean sheets felt, I had a nagging paranoia about my health and being somewhat on my own, without a nursing staff to care for me. I didn't truly need them, as Barb was taking good care of me, but I felt uneasy and concerned that I might have an issue or an episode at home that I wouldn't be prepared for. I felt vulnerable and insecure in an unfamiliar way.

I shared my concerns with Barb and told her that I felt a bit like her brothers, both of whom had had heart stent surgery in the past months. I feared I might have a problem in my sleep, possibly another stroke. She listened and reassured me that my situation was very different from theirs. Yes, I had a stent, but all my arteries were clean and free of plaque. I was not a candidate for another stroke, and I should relax. I thanked her and we kissed, then held each other. And then I went to sleep—in my own bed, without the use of Percocet.

My New Daily Routine and First Day Home (April 9, 2008)

I used to wake up and do stretches and push-ups in the den for twenty minutes before heading down to my home office for a good four to five hours of typing, reading, and phone calls. This morning was a bit different. I had slept in my T-shirt, so I wouldn't have to try to dress myself, but I struggled mightily with the sweatpants as I guided them on with one hand; all in all, not *too* bad. I went to the den to start my routine, but instead of stretching and push-ups, I practiced picking up small items and doing finger exercises with my putty, all the while staring longingly at my guitar. It's not that I wasn't able to stretch my body; I just didn't have the will.

I'm a morning person. Ever since I started working in the dry cleaning business, I've woken up at five o'clock in the morning, without the aid of coffee or an alarm clock. I normally move like a whirling dervish, with all kinds of mental and physical energy until around 5 PM when I start to wind down, and I usually crash hard around 10.

This morning, on my first day home from the hospital, I was feeling lethargic and out of sorts in so many ways, though I was excited to be *doing* something. I did my exercises, watching more TV than usual, and waited for Barb to get up. Making breakfast was, unfortunately, not in the realm of possibility. Yes, my right hand was 75 percent useful, but my own body felt foreign to me, and my left side was still basically useless.

I don't know what I thought life would be like once I was home, but I had been terribly mistaken if I thought there would be some semblance of normality.

Since Barb still had a few hours more to sleep, I decided to try to work through some of the backlog in the office. I walked into my sanctuary downstairs—the "command center" as I call it. I opened the blinds, looked at the sun-splashed mountains, let out an audible cry of happiness to be home, and dug in. I began by organizing the bills and documents on my desk. The stroke had affected my cognitive abilities and capacity to think in an orderly manner, and it took me ten minutes to sort through all the paper. Then I stared at them for a few more minutes. This was going to be a huge challenge.

I lit up the computer screen by clicking the mouse, using my right hand to some effect. My brain function was basically equal to my one-finger pecking, so there was actually some poetry in motion (albeit slow motion). I went back to my email, which I'd tried to sort the night before. The lines, words, and folders looked jumbled and unclear. I had the hardest time seeing the words, comprehending their meaning, and deciphering one line from the next. I tried magnifying glasses to ease my vision problems but they didn't help, because the problem wasn't just my vision—my brain couldn't turn the letters into anything meaningful.

About seven years earlier I had started an online business to complement my writing and consulting. The release of my first book had brought me to national attention. I'd gotten some speaking gigs at conventions, had done some one-on-one consulting with dry cleaners, and had given hundreds of interviews to magazines, newspapers, and radio shows. After a lot of work and some well-placed phone calls I was invited to be a guest on ABC's *The View* with Barbara Walters. Barb and Ben came to New York with me and watched the live show from the sidelines.

The exposure from this and other national shows, along with the magazine interviews, had begun to make The Clothing Doctor a household name. It also helped build a growing online business—hence the backlog of email, online store orders, and phone calls to return when I got back from the hospital.

I am nothing if not stubborn and driven, so I used my finger and a metal ruler to follow the words on the computer screen, word by word, line by line, as I read and deleted junk mail. I was backlogged and frustrated, but I kept plugging away. If I'd had an angel looking over my shoulder, it would have insisted that I stop pushing so hard and just freaking rest. It was my first full day back, and I had to chill out! The therapist and Dr. Zacharias had warned me about fatigue and suggested that I acclimate slowly once I got home. I had spent almost two hours futzing and pushing papers, with some positive results. But I was beat, and it was only 9:00 a.m.

I went back upstairs and kissed Barb good morning. I mentioned the work I'd been doing, and she scolded me.

"You have to rest and take it easy. There's plenty of time to get back to people and to do business. You have to pace yourself."

She was absolutely correct, as she often is. Barb would be gone most of the day, taking her dance classes and running errands, doing twice the work. We discussed her plans for the day, which included filling my prescription for Plavix—my first goddamn pharmaceutical, other than an antibiotic when I was a kid.

I went to lie down on the sofa and fell asleep in moments. This late morning/early afternoon nap would become a regular routine for many months to come. I would wake a few hours later feeling a little out of it, but with renewed energy— and it would take all the energy I could muster to cope with the changes in my post-stroke life.

Chapter 10

THE EASIEST THINGS
MADE DIFFICULT

Life at home used to look like this: After my morning exercises and the requisite hours in front of the computer, I'd do the dishes and then throw on some clothing for tennis, hiking, rollerblading, a dance movement class, or skiing in the winter. I'd drive into town to run errands, possibly catch some lunch—sometimes with Barb—then drive back up to the house and do a few chores. Then I'd play guitar until Barb got home. We'd decide on dinner and possibly take in a movie, or read the paper and do the crossword puzzle— one of Barb's passions, with me contributing when I could. On weekends we'd often eat out, maybe followed by some live music and dancing with friends. Being in our fifties, with our sons out of the house, we were free to do whatever we wanted.

But hold it! That was then, and this was now—a whole new ballgame.

Home for just a few days, my lifestyle was far from what I was used to, but filled nonetheless with a myriad of time-consuming tasks. It started with shaving. The first time I looked in the mirror to shave, I did not look like I remembered; my face was less friendly and less relaxed, more angular; my hair looked like it belonged to someone else, with different waves governed by a mind of its own. My vision was skewed and I couldn't focus. I asked Barb for her opinion, but she said that I looked the same as before.

Back in the days of my radio show, I got the chance to interview Klaus Obermeyer, the famed pioneer and maker of Obermeyer Skiwear, and the inventor of the first down jacket. Klaus was eighty-six years old at the time, but he still skied every day. I asked him how he'd remained so vital and young at heart. In his lilting Austrian accent, he answered, "I feel the same as I did when I was young. I look in the mirror to shave and I say to myself, 'I don't know you, but I shave you anyway!'"

I felt like I was shaving someone else's face those first days. With a shaky razor and a dead left hand, I hacked away, nicking myself often. It took months for my face to once again look familiar and friendly.

I wasted no time scheduling my first rehab appointments. Between physical therapy, occupational therapy, speech therapy, and acupuncture, my dance card was filled. The rehab center blended speech therapy with occupational therapy (OT). Since I could speak clearly and only struggled with choosing the right words, my course of therapy was mostly occupational. I had two hours of OT almost every day, followed by acupuncture. I was excited to start the healing, but distressed that Barb would have to drive me to all these appointments. If you want to emasculate a man fast, just take away his car and driving privileges.

I dressed in loose pullover shirts since buttons were out of the question. I needed help pulling them over my head and couldn't get my arms in the sleeves without assistance. I wore sweatpants because I couldn't operate the zipper on my beloved jeans with one hand. Putting on socks was another challenge, but it was too cold to go without them. I pulled with my right hand, three or four times in each direction, to get the sock on each foot, yanking, straightening, and finally evening the toe area so it didn't bunch up inside the shoe. I wore slip-on shoes, but they still required some work to get on. Getting

my wallet into the zip pocket of my fleece sweatshirt took another few minutes. Getting out the door on time would prove
to be a major roadblock for close to a year.

My First Therapy Sessions – OT

On my second day home, Barb dropped me off at the Boulder
Center for Neurologic and Orthopedic Rehabilitation. Fortunately it was just a short drive down the mountain. The facility was situated at the base of the foothills, with views of the
mountains from the rehab room. I walked into the building
and immediately smelled the familiar scent of an indoor swimming pool. I had been on the swim team for most of my ado-
lescent and teen years and practiced indoor during the winter
season, so that moist chlorine smell always brought back
memories.

As I passed the swimming pool on my way to the registra-
tion desk, I could see people in the pool doing physical therapy
(PT). I thought that would be the perfect place to rehab my
body and shoulder. The double doors had a handicap button
to open them automatically, but I used the opportunity to test
myself. It hurt my shoulder to swing them open, and it took
some strength, but I got it.

I found the desk and checked in. This entailed the kind of
small motor skills that reduced me to early childhood. I spent
a full minute fumbling to get my wallet out of my pocket, and
then some frustrating moments trying to dig out my insurance
card. Then another minute or so more to get the card back in
the wallet and the zipper closed.

I was given the obligatory clipboard and pen to answer
pages of questions. Reading was the hard part. Writing was
easier, but still not a breeze. My cognitive ability was hampered and cloudy, so understanding the questions took time
and made me anxious. I looked around the waiting room to

see who was in worse shape than me—which seems to be a common game people play at doctors' offices and hospitals. I could also see inside one of the rehab rooms, so I watched the therapy process while I waited my turn. A few people moved with crutches and canes. Some wore neck braces, slings, and such. Everybody—men, women, and kids—was there to regain the use of part of their body and/or brain; to *relearn* something.

My occupational therapist, Mary, was a woman of about forty, cheerful and attractive, with long blonde hair and an easy, welcoming demeanor. She offered me water, and we chatted in her office as she reviewed my records. We talked about the whole experience, and she asked me specific questions about my lifestyle: what I did for fun, what chores I did at home, what kind of sports I played, if any. She wanted to know what kind of work I did, with all the details—heavy lifting, typing, handiwork—so she could assess how difficult it would be for me during the coming year. Was I dependent on work for money, or did I have some savings? Would I collect disability, since I was not able to work at the capacity I had before? Was Barb available to help me, and was she supportive?

I knew that Mary must have heard all kinds of stories sadder and more severe than mine. I found the questions kind of personal and a bit odd, as it was all new to me. She saw the puzzled look on my face and explained: she needed all these details because she was interested in my life as a whole and how I was going to cope with my day-to-day challenges, mentally and physically. She already knew, from her years of experience, what it had taken for me to get dressed and out the door that morning. We spent most of our time the first day reviewing these minute details and getting to know each other. It was like visiting a shrink, but more interesting.

Mary told me to relax and take things easy for a while. I needed to understand that therapy, both at the rehab center and at home, would be very draining, and I should pay careful attention to my mind and body. I would need ample breaks and extra nap time. When I felt overwhelmed or overloaded, I should take a break.

"Do *not* push through it," she instructed.

I thought of my ill-fated morning in the command center and resolved to take her—and Barb's—advice.

We did some baseline tests to evaluate the severity of my disabilities. These tests would determine my visual processing speed. I had three minutes for each test. She gave me a sheet with one-, two-, and three-digit numbers running across the page in a line, and it was my job to identify and circle the numbers in each row that contained the same numerals: 61 and 16; 14 and 41; 452 and 542, etc. This test would hopefully help reveal the extent of my recent trouble identifying and understanding numbers.

The next test was much longer and featured a series of pictures — twenty-two per page. There were images of a soccer ball, a cup of coffee, and a puppy dog. I had to circle the pairs; wherever there was a cup of coffee and a puppy together, side by side. They were small images, and there were so many that I began seeing double. I found this work overwhelming and stressful. (As I was writing this entry today, five months later, I proofed the word "stressful" and noticed that I'd missed the first "s"—*the leftmost letter!*)

The last test for the day examined my cognitive abilities in an exercise that dealt with decision speed. The pages contained rows of six images, and I had to find the two that were most related or most alike. A sample row contained a round clock with hands, a comb, an envelope, a nail, a hat, and a digital clock. In this case, it was the two clocks that were similar. Pretty simple, huh? I did better on these. The following pages were trickier and contained more images with more obscure likenesses, such as a half moon, a dog, a star, and an umbrella.

This was one of the most strenuous tests I'd taken, and I was very confused. I did these tests for a few weeks, and among a national group of "normal" fifty-three-year-olds, I scored in the fifth percentile. In other words, 95 percent of those tested did better than me.

By the end of our time that day, Mary could tell that I was driven and impatient, which could work both for me and against me. Yes, stubborn people like me do tend to heal quicker and get back to daily routines faster, but they also tend to be more fatigued, which can have a negative effect. I appreciated Mary's soft-spoken approach and took her advice to heart. I'd see her in two days for our next session. I had the feeling that we would become quite close in the coming months.

My First Physical Therapy

Mary led me to the physical therapy room and introduced me to Karen. The room held all kinds of therapeutic apparatus and doodads. Karen, a sturdy woman in her forties, asked me to sit on a padded table. She adjusted the height of the table with a hydraulic foot pedal until I was even with the work tray.

We'd start, she explained, by testing my hand-grip strength and then finger strength, both of which I would need to regain in order to relearn those everyday motions like buttoning and zipping. All of these tests would be administered on both hands to determine baseline readings for my condition, and then we'd compare them with my readings in three months. I will share these numbers for my left hand only, as that was the most affected:

Hand Grip Strength: 79 pounds pressure
Thumb & One Finger: 10 pounds
Thumb & Two Fingers: 18 pounds

Needless to say, my scores were well below normal for a healthy person.

Next was the 9-Hole Peg Test. I was given a Tupperware-type container with twenty small wooden dowels in it. The dowels were about two inches long and narrower than a pencil. I had to reach into the container, pick up one dowel at a time, and place each one into a block of wood with drilled holes. It seemed pretty easy; then again, it also seems like it would be easy to finish a twenty-two ounce steak when you're starving. But having the desire isn't always enough.

Karen asked me to start with my left hand and she clicked the stopwatch. I had a very hard time getting my hand into the container; it seemed too small. I finally guided my hand into the container and tried to grasp a dowel. I did not have the ability to grasp a single one. In all fairness, my left hand felt numb and thick—as bloated as a Mickey Mouse glove. Due to my inability to pronate my hand, position it directly into the container, and control my finger response, I struggled until we reached the one-minute mark and she clicked the timer to stop it. I had picked up zero, zilch, not even one dowel over the course of a full minute.

Karen gently explained, "While your performance did not produce positive results, it did establish a baseline reading. You shouldn't be too upset. On the positive side, it can only get better, and you *will* get better."

My next challenge, the One-Minute Block Test, involved a wooden box with a tray on each side. I had to lift a one-inch-square wooden cube out of the box and then throw it into the empty tray next to it, without causing it to bounce out. I did a little better this time; the blocks were larger and easier to grasp than the dreaded dowels. My score: 19 blocks in 60 seconds.

While I did a good deal better with my right hand on both tests, my scores were still below the normal benchmark for an average healthy person.

The next tests measured my visual tracking and peripheral awareness. These exercises judged how well I could adjust to close, middle, and faraway text and images.

I would look at Karen's nose, and then she would hold up a single finger to the left and right to see if I could see both in my periphery, while still looking at her nose. The results:

> Tracking: Decreased awareness—very slow moving left to right.
> Peripheral: Decreased performance—severe "left field vision cut."

This is why I missed the "B" in "Brain" on that hospital poster—and why I still wasn't allowed to drive myself.

Once Karen understood the extent of my problem, she emphasized that although it was bad, it would get better with some exercises and with time. We talked about corrective lenses and how they work, if it turned out that I needed them. She gave me a list of items to work on at home, which concluded my first day of OT and PT.

On my day off from therapy I did the exercises I'd been given. I started them in the morning and did them through-out the day and night as I was able. I had my first acupuncture appointment that afternoon. I've used acupuncture for many years to treat migraine headaches, various sports injuries, and for general wellness, with positive results. I had been told that acupuncture was good for stroke survivors—that it should be good for nerve regeneration and stimulation in my damaged limbs and throughout my body—so I had high expectations.

I told Livia, our acupuncturist, about the stroke and conveyed as best as I could how my left hand felt "thick." She treated me, and when I got off the table, I noticed an immediate change in the thickness. I made the best fist I could muster, and it felt thinner.

By the time Barb picked me up, though, my hand had returned to the way it felt before, thick and stiff. And even though I had slept on the table—as I've always done—I was totally worn out by the session and took a long nap when I got home. When I woke, I was still extremely drained, weak, and lethargic. Still, I was hopeful that the acupuncture treatments would complement and help accelerate my recovery.

Chapter 11

BACK TO BUSINESS

Passover (Two Weeks Home)

This year Barb and I were invited to observe Passover with friends in Boulder, our first Seder since moving away from the DC area. Although it felt way too soon to go out to a busy event with lots of people, I went anyway. After all, I am Jewish, and Passover Seder is a tradition. It would be very low-key, with only nine guests. We met several new people, then gathered around the table.

Our friend Alice had photocopied a number of her favorite readings, along with many of the standard passages. As the host, she called on people to read, moving around the table. She had thoughtfully supplied a pair of "magnifiers" to pass around for the older folks like Barb and me.

I felt uncertain about reading, but eager to try. When my turn came, I slipped on my reading glasses and began. I read very slowly, but with confidence. I would envision the words and then enunciate them as clearly and evenly as I could. After I finished my section, people around the table looked at me kind of strangely.

Barb was the first to speak. "Did you know that you missed the first word of every sentence?"

I hadn't noticed that, but I understood how it was entirely possible. If the Seder book had been written in Hebrew, I would have read it from right to left, and instead missed the words at the *end* of the sentence (that is, if I actually read Hebrew!).

Until that point, the guests hadn't known about my stroke—we only chatted a little before the Seder, and my speech had been normal—so they were a bit shocked by my reading troubles. Soon, I found myself explaining to them all about my stroke and my current disabilities. It was the first time I'd spoken about it in public, but I felt comfortable, which put the others at ease in what could have been an awkward moment. I welcomed the ensuing questions and openly shared a bit of my story.

In the end all were supportive, and I felt grateful to be celebrating another Passover.

A Humbling Experience (Three Weeks After the Stroke)

I was told to judge my improvement in terms of months and even years, but each day was a new day, with new challenges and discoveries. Just as new parents count a newborn baby's life in days and then weeks, I counted my new life in small steps. Each day was long, and filled with tasks that took forever. From getting dressed, to doing therapy, to picking up one single tablet of Plavix each morning—everything was a chore, and everything took longer than anticipated. I have a friend my age in Boulder who suffered a debilitating stroke when she was in her twenties, and she spends a good part of her days on simple activities like dressing and making meals, so I know how lucky I am.

I decided that this was the day to plow through the ten or so orders we had filled and shipped from the online store during and prior to my hospital stay. I had to match credit card and PayPal charges to invoices, and then enter the data on a spreadsheet. I'd been dreading this process, but wanted to see what I could actually do.

The computer presented the most intense and demanding mental work I'd done since the stroke, and it was brutal. It was way too early in my rehabilitation for me to be tackling such a task, and I knew this. I understood from the initial tests in the ICU that my cognitive abilities were diminished, but my ability to verbally organize my thoughts gave me a false sense of confidence. Nevertheless, reading was extremely difficult with the left field vision cut, and my comprehension of the written word was severely hampered. To read and comprehend incisively would come—but I wasn't there yet. I forged ahead anyway.

Switching back and forth from the spreadsheet to the email inbox to the paper invoices meant that I had to refocus my eyes on a specific line, on each document, many times over, when I was still having problems doing it even once without severe anxiety and fatigue. I am stubborn, though in this case some may say stupid, but I couldn't sit by and watch the work mount up. Mary's words from OT echoed in my head: "Rest as much as possible and *do not overdo it*. There's no gain in overworking at this stage in your recovery. Less is more." Not exactly my mantra. In my pre-stroke days, this pile of work would have taken fifteen minutes, max.

The project was pure torture. I used a ruler to help me read the lines, but my head still spun and whirled for minutes on end, every time my eyes switched documents. Each time I refocused, it took additional minutes to readjust my vision to the page or the screen. The numbers on the spreadsheet all ran together, and I repeatedly entered numbers on the wrong lines, which caused a cumulative effect down the spreadsheet, affecting every previous entry. Even when I *could* make out the numbers, I could barely comprehend what I was seeing. I tried changing the font style and increasing the size to be large enough for a seeing-impaired person to read it, but it didn't make a difference.

It took me over two hours to do fifteen minutes' worth of work. I did ultimately accomplish the task, but I walked away feeling like I'd lost a battle, and with a whole new re-spect for my condition. I dragged myself from the command center to the den and collapsed onto the couch for a long and much-needed restorative nap. From this point on, Barb read my emails aloud, and made all the computer entries for me. I found I was becoming more patient with others and myself.

The Continuing Saga (Almost Four Weeks)

I committed myself to rehabilitation and would stop at noth-ing until I got my faculties back. Each day was filled with PT and OT, acupuncture, and hours of practicing my exercises on my own. The therapists impressed this upon me from the start: I was the master of my own destiny. Yes, I could only heal to the degree that my body and mind would allow; I could not fool Mother Nature. But *everything* outside of that—therapy at rehab, therapy at home, my constant vigilance and commit-ment on an hourly and daily basis—was in my control. It was time to be strong and to put my mind, body, and will where my mouth was. I wanted it all back. So I went to therapy and I did my homework, as boring and repetitive as it often was.

My next session with Mary was again a sobering one: another reminder of where I was and how far I had to go. We talked for the first twenty minutes, as was our routine, assessing my skills. Then she had me play a computer game, in which I had to capture or tag objects as they floated across the screen, in some cases dragging them into a folder or box. I struggled to follow and click the objects; my eyes simply couldn't keep up.

Mary explained that stroke survivors and rehab patients always want immediate gratification and fast results, and are often in denial about their deficits. Health care profession-als and therapists consider a week—or even a month—to be nothing, a mere blip in the scope of rehabilitation. The survivor, on the other hand, perceives this time in slow motion. Mary felt that I was acutely aware of my deficits, which is a huge plus for people with frontal lobe issues and injuries. Because I had good insight, I was able to move on and do the work. Being an athlete and having extra leisure time for rehab were additional factors that worked in my favor in this game of balancing work, rehab, and play.

Next, as a verbal and cognitive test, Mary listed five items and had me repeat them. Then she listed six, and then seven. I did pretty well on the fives and okay on the sixes, but I burned out millions of brain cells trying to recite back the sevens. I kept a positive attitude, but when I finished I was licked.

Physical therapy, however, was right up my alley. Karen would introduce new tests and games at each visit, so the sessions held my interest. On this particular day we went to the rehab gym to address my frozen shoulder. I was having real issues with strength and range of motion. Anything above my head was impossible to reach.

Karen gave me some strengthening exercises using light barbells, such as one-hand rows, curls, and arm lifts. She also had me work with a Thera-band®, a flat, five-inch-wide rubber band that comes in different tensions identified by color, with yellow being the lightest and easiest. I knew the Thera-band® from Pilates; we had them all over our house.

Back on the padded work table in the office, she had me lie on my back with my arm extended as far as possible behind my head. The position was painful, so she warned me to listen to my body. Karen gradually added weight to the extended arm to increase the stretch. This was good; the workout resonated with me. She also gave me a tool called a Digi-Flex, for strengthening and isolating each finger, which I took home to add to my collection of PT toys. I left the session with a slew of new things to practice.

Chapter 12

MY HANDS!

May 2008, About Five Weeks

My den, which had always been a room for relaxation, guitar-playing, afternoon naps, and movies at night, was starting to look like a rehab center and became a constant reminder of my condition. I tried to maintain a positive attitude toward life and the work ahead of me, but at times I felt overwhelmed, impatient, and defeated.

I had a small wicker basket filled with chrome "Chinese balls," hot-pink therapy putty, the Digi-Flex, and a tennis ball to hold and squeeze. The Chinese balls, which sounded like musical bells, were a recent addition. I had used a set with Karen during PT the week before, and she suggested that I buy my own. The idea is to hold both of the little metal balls in one hand, with one ball cradled in the first digits of the fingertips and the other in the center of the palm, and to slowly and silently move them in a circular motion, without clanking them together. I started by moving them in the easier, more natural direction, and then in the other. I had a hard time doing it in both directions with my right hand and couldn't even do one direction with my left. Nonetheless, I resolved to keep using them as another way to gauge my improvement.

During the endless hours of practice, I began to fantasize about becoming ambidextrous, or at least a lot less gimpy with my left hand. I wanted to close the huge gap between my left-handed and right-handed skills. It would require a sizable commitment in terms of time and will, but just the thought of becoming better at something than I was before the stroke was appealing, even in my diminished capacity.

By May my body was coming around, albeit slowly, and my days had taken on a predictable routine: outpatient therapy during the day, practice at home in the afternoon, and a movie at night. I was growing bored and frustrated being home all the time, unable to drive, unable to play tennis, and not yet surefooted enough to take walks or to hike the trails near our house. I knew it would all take time, but I was impatient, and my impatience led to a bit of depression.

My left hand was the bane of my life. I could not carry a glass of water or a plate in that hand without spilling it. I could not pour myself a glass of water. And I still couldn't form the chords to play guitar.

The paralysis had left my hand in a C-shaped "claw" that rendered it basically useless. I spent time every day unfurling my fingers from the claw position, stretching them, strengthening them, and massaging them, and took every opportunity to use the hand. I could actually lift my glass during dinner with the left hand but, because of the claw shape, I could not release the glass without a considerable amount of attention. Even then, due to the numbness, I didn't always sense if I had actually released my grasp on the glass when I put it down, which sometimes led to spills.

There's a poignant scene from the movie, *Regarding Henry*, after he returns from months in a rehab hospital. He and his daughter and wife are sitting at the kitchen table when his daughter accidentally spills her orange juice. She's a very responsible kid, so she's embarrassed about it. Henry looks at her with a crooked, paralysis-induced smile and says, "That's okay, honey, I do that all the time," and then he intentionally knocks his glass over, too. His daughter laughs with delight, but his wife and housekeeper are horrified that this former type A power lawyer has fallen so far.

Looking for compassion and empathy, I reminded Barb of that scene after I knocked over my glass—again. She was more understanding about the spill than I was. I kept my sense of humor about it, but I still felt embarrassed.

It is one thing to have severely diminished ability and performance when doing a solitary task with *just* your left hand, but let's not forget that the left hand is also a willing and necessary participant in all two-handed endeavors, such as zipping and buttoning, pulling up pants, washing dishes, typing, applying toothpaste, tying shoelaces . . . the list goes on. If you doubt me, try holding your nondominant hand behind your back when you first get up in the morning and notice how many processes you probably take for granted, day after day.

My hand was still numb, which made everything that much harder. For example, I had trouble placing my wallet in my pocket. I've always worn it in my back left pocket, so I naturally used my left hand to slide it into the pocket and remove it. Rather than reaching across my back with my right hand, which felt awkward, I tried to make it work with my left hand anyway, considering the effort to be another form of therapy. I like playing games, so this new challenge would act as another gauge by which to judge my improvement.

Recovery is all about forging new neural pathways and finding new ways to do old things. The nerve damage from stroke often erases many of the old pathways that were used to perform these tasks, many of which we learned way back as children. I do not presume even for a moment to suggest that my ailment begins to compare to the challenges of people with permanent disabilities, but I definitely have more understanding and compassion for them now.

That week I experienced some computer problems. I called tech support, who guided me through the troubleshooting process, but I was still having trouble. When I couldn't even plug my laptop back into its docking station with my good hand, I finally gave in and explained things to the guy on the phone.

"This is not your problem at all," I said, "and I hate to concern you with this, but I had a stroke recently so I'm almost learning-disabled; I'll need you to repeat some things. At the moment, I cannot seem to get the computer back into the docking station."

To my surprise, he told me, "My grandmother lived with us for many years, and toward the end of her life she had a stroke, so I understand what you're going through. There's no hurry. Just relax."

I felt genuinely touched and very relieved, and I thanked him for understanding. However, at that moment, I had the strange realization that I was, in fact, "disabled," which really floored me. I thought for a moment, and recognized that it was time to truly accept my disability. By admitting to my condition, I could now move forward and rethink the challenge at hand.

Admitting my fallibility may have helped set me free, but the docking station was really unnerving me. I studied the laptop and the docking station for a full minute, trying to figure out what I was missing. Then I remembered the left field cut in my vision. Everything I looked at was skewed. So I simply moved the laptop over about one inch, and it clicked right in. Between my slow brain, my inability to reason, and my vision problem, I'd completely missed the cues. We rebooted the computer, and—voilà!—It worked.

Chapter 13

GOOD DAYS AND
BAD DAYS

My Daily Routine (Six Weeks)

My sessions with Karen became a lifeline for me. Each hour we spent together produced positive results, along with some growing frustration. I would go into PT with new issues, and she'd introduce a new type of therapy to address them. My vision and my hands were ongoing problems, so we'd do reading and eye control exercises for half the time and shoulder strengthening and hand coordination the other half.

We studied sign language, which required considerable finger isolation and dexterity. This was a particularly challenging exercise because my hand still had the claw thing going. Moving each finger into place was a slow, meticulous process, and I used my relatively good right hand to help position my gimpy left hand. We started with the letter A, which required me to hold my palm forward vertically while bending four fingers forward to touch the palm of my hand, almost like making a fist. The arduous process of getting each finger into position was fantastic therapy. We made our way through the alphabet and—as painstaking as it was—I really enjoyed it. I found the letter "U" to be one of the hardest because I had to uncurl two fingers of my claw. At home I would practice the sign language movements until I became totally fatigued.

As a final exercise we touched on "saccadic eye movement," rapid eye movements left and right, back and forth. For this we played volleyball with an inflated balloon, which really tested my abilities to follow an object and then hit it. The game also tested my eye-hand coordination.

In an attempt to help around the house and to continue branching out, I started washing dishes again. I always hold the item in my left hand and wash with my right. But with my left hand unable to feel the glass or dish I was holding, the chore took a long time to complete. The first night I attempted it, Barb had made a fantastic meal, so I had about fifteen pieces to wash, in all shapes and sizes. I put a padded rubber mat in the sink to help steady the glasses and dishes, and to prevent breakage. I held onto each soapy dish and glass as if it were the finest crystal and began scrubbing. Barb offered to help, but I insisted that I do it on my own.

The process was slow and laborious, and even more difficult than I imagined. It took over twenty minutes, but it felt good and I was proud of myself. Over the next few weeks, I took over dishwashing duties. I ended up breaking one glass and a bowl, but it was definitely the right time to get back to this chore.

I continued to "play" guitar, even though I could hardly play a clear, ringing note. I started with very simple groups of notes and worked hard to try to form a D-chord. Bar chords require a firm, controlled left hand to depress all six strings at once, but it would take a lot more therapy and healing before I could get there.

An Epiphany, Shall We Say?

I had kept a positive attitude from the moment I had the stroke and got the diagnosis, but after four or five weeks of intense therapy and acupuncture, I hit a wall. I was depressed about my limited lifestyle, my physical disabilities, and my inability to drive, and I developed a raging case of cabin fever. This led to a growing frustration and overall dissatisfaction with life. I was accustomed to daily physical exercise and sports that moved my blood, and I sorely missed the endorphin rush that accompanies sports and the high I get from performing, competing, and perspiring. I was losing my interest in rehab and I still had untold months of it ahead of me. I still felt reluctant to take antidepressants; the last thing I wanted was to be on another drug in addition to Plavix.

I'd been a good boy ever since I left the hospital; no alcohol, no partying—not that I felt much like socializing or drinking. Dr. Zacharias had told me not to drink. As a creative guy with a penchant for new experiences, I had smoked pot at different times in my life. I've used it as a catalyst when I've been creatively blocked in my writing, music, and business life. I've also used it to relax and space out after a particularly shitty day at work. The stroke had made me permanently spacey, however, so I wouldn't need reefer for that!

On one particular day, I was fed up with everything and needed an escape. I decided to take a single hit of pot to see what that could do for me. I spent quite a bit of time on the Internet researching potential complications from taking Plavix and smoking pot. I found no mention of any, but I did read that marijuana was considered to be a blood thinner, which is what Plavix does, so I concluded that I was safe. Left to my own devices and with Barb out every day, it sounded like a good approach at this particularly tough time. I was desperate for a change.

My experiment yielded instant results. I took one drag on my little pipe, and within ten minutes I was in the living room trying to juggle three tennis balls. Of course I couldn't actually juggle, although I had been good at it prior to the stroke. Juggling requires a series of fast catch-and-release movements as the ball transfers from hand to hand. You have to walk before you can run, so I broke the process down step-by-step. Next, I tried juggling just two balls in my left hand—one ball going up and one ball coming down. Still no success. Then I decided that all I wanted to do was catch the ball, and forget the juggling. I simplified the process even more by just tossing one ball up with my right hand and catching it with my left. When the ball landed in my gimpy left hand, however, I wasn't able to grab the ball to close the deal.

I repeated the toss-and-catch process many times, observing the problems and making adjustments. I needed to use both my palm and my fingers to trap the ball in my hand. The main problem was opening and closing the hand fast enough to catch, release, and toss. I could get the hand open, but closing it and letting go was much more challenging.

By breaking down the process and repeating it, I realized, I would forge a new neural pathway for catching the ball. It was only a matter of time. I spent ten minutes on this pursuit, chasing the ball every time it fell to the floor and rolled away. This was the most movement and the most fun I'd had since the stroke. If the reefer turned me into a child for an hour, then so be it.

Even though I could not juggle, the point of all this was not lost. Smoking a little pot pulled me out of my malaise and gave me the emotional break I needed from the day-in, day-out drudgery of therapy and practice. I was trapped in my physical body and could not get out on my own—or perhaps I couldn't get *into* my body and out of my brain?

Smoking helped me escape the confines of my "stroked" body and get back in touch with it. It altered my perception of myself as a stroke survivor and presented a host of new possibilities that I could not envision while being "stuck" in my physical body. The pot boosted my spirits, restored my normally upbeat sense of humor, reenergized me, and gave me the strength to stay on a positive path, moving forward. For the first time since the stroke I felt a connection to my physical body. I was a new man.

I know this is a rather unorthodox approach, and probably frowned upon by the medical profession (even though medical marijuana is legal in Colorado), but I didn't care. Let the experts experience a stroke, with all of its side effects and symptoms, and then tell me that what I was doing was wrong. Granted, I do not necessarily endorse or condone this for every stroke victim, but it did something very positive for me.

Freeing my body to chase the balls—and being able to laugh about it—was a gift. But perhaps just as important was learning to recognize and accept the work and the fundamentals necessary to forge new pathways in the brain. A stroke is a brain injury, after all, and the brain needs to adapt and heal. I had to break down the processes of catching a ball, just as I had done with every other newly acquired skill. I put two and two together, and that in itself was a victory.

The Long Road Back (Seven Weeks)

I took my guitar with me to PT to show Karen the problems I was having fingering notes. I asked her to watch my fingers and hand position as I tried to form them into a D-chord. My fingers shook as I tried to position and press them flat against the fret board of the guitar. If they do not lie flat on the strings, then the sound becomes muffled. My fingers felt arthritic and would not respond to the message from my brain.

Karen observed me as I tried to form the chord, and then we talked about it. She suggested that I use the Digi-Flex tool she had given me to strengthen and isolate finger movements. A while back she'd also given me an exercise involving newspaper. The idea was to take a quarter page of newspaper and, with just my left hand, slowly crush it into a ball in the palm of my hand. If I did both these exercises, and worked hard at it, I should gain the dexterity to finger the D-chord properly— once I could supinate my hand. I needed to be able to lay my hand flat on a table, palm down, before I could properly form chords on the guitar.

When I attempted to lay my left hand palm down, however, the thumb would ride up and curl about an inch off the tabletop. This was the same dilemma that caused water to spill over the left side of my glass.

I suggested to Karen that the problem stemmed from my frozen left shoulder—that my inability to get that part of my body into the proper position made my hand unable to properly supinate. I felt that this was the bigger problem, and she concurred. This decision led to a new exercise that would help realign my shoulder turn.

I left PT with homework that I hoped would do the trick, but it would take a lot of work and focus, some of which would likely be very painful. Karen always warned me about stopping all exercises just short of pain and discomfort. But I still maintained "No pain, no gain." We agreed to disagree, and I left her office feeling good about the latest challenge.

Over the next few days, I worked hard in the command center and in the den. At some point that week, I had a setback that scared me. My vision was off, my hand shook, and I was feeling out of sorts. My shoulder and hand were still stiff and numb, which I was used to, but this felt bizarre and more severe. I thought I might be having another TIA or a ministroke.

I stopped into PT without an appointment to see if Karen could see me on the fly. After I described my sensations, we repeated the peg-in-the-hole test and some vision stuff, and she confirmed that I was slower and less focused. This was bad news, and I had no safety net to catch me. She suggested that I go see Dr. Zacharias as soon as possible.

Fortunately, Dr. Zacharias had an opening that day. He tested my reflexes and coordination. He told me that everything was fine, but that I should remember that recovery is long and often uneven, and that there would be days like this.

The next day I felt much better, with no lingering effects in my shoulder, hand, or vision. The symptoms went away as quickly as they appeared.

That night, Barb and I went to see my friend, Erik Deutsch, perform with his band at a local coffeehouse. When I'd dressed for the evening, I had made a semi-conscious decision to wear my jeans with the button-down fly, instead of a zippered pair. It took me the better part of three minutes to button them, but I figured it would be good therapy. Barb saw me struggling and offered to help, but I insisted on doing it myself. Still, Barb assured me that if I needed any help in the restroom that evening, she would be there for me. After a bottle of water and a Chai tea during the show, it was time to go. I excused myself from the table and, as naturally as possible, ambled to the back of the room. Both bathrooms were full and there was a line, which concerned me a bit. I am a normal fifty-something man with a healthy prostate, but when I have to go, I have to go. By the time I got in, I really had to pee.

I stood in front of the toilet and began unbuttoning my pants. I undid the top waist button rather easily, with five more to go. I hummed and whistled as I struggled with the fly buttons, from top to bottom. This was becoming tricky. I began to tense up, which didn't help my dexterity or my bladder. I stammered, swore, and cursed myself for being so stupid. I even danced in place: anything and everything to occupy my mind while I wrestled with the resistant buttons.

Like the last moments of a dream before waking, when twenty things happen at once, the situation was growing more intense and more desperate by the second. What had started as a simple challenge and another game quickly turned into a very uncomfortable experience. The moments turned into minutes, and my stress turned into recrimination. I began to sweat and curse myself. It was a damn good thing that I was alone, because I must have looked like an idiot.

In the closing seconds, I did, ultimately, relieve myself, but it took a long time for me to stop hyperventilating. Looking in the mirror as I washed my hands, I saw a childish fool, albeit a victorious one.

Chapter 14

IT'S TIME TO DRIVE!

I was closing in on eight weeks after the stroke, and I sensed that it was time to get behind the wheel. I pulled my car out of the garage and drove a hundred feet up our private road. It felt strange to drive and even more strange to be alone in the car, but I also felt independent and grown up.

My spatial awareness was a bit skewed due to my vision. I drove to the first switchback above my house and maneuvered the car into reverse to turn back to our garage. Besides the somewhat bizarre feeling of driving, my biggest challenge was trying to turn the steering wheel with my frozen shoulder. It hurt like hell to steer, which worried me a little as I thought about driving in traffic. Nevertheless, as I re-parked the car in the garage, I knew that I would be driving again very soon.

I was feeling better on many fronts. In preparation for greater independence and my pending return to driving, I decided to begin working out at a gym. Barb took me to the North Boulder Recreation Center at the bottom of the mountain, and I went to the weight room. I was determined to loosen up my shoulder with some light lifting.

First I did some stretches, using the apparatus as counterpoint and support. Although I was moving my body in a familiar way, the motions felt otherworldly. I did lifts targeting legs, arms, and some chest, doing three sets of each with moderate weight. I also used some of the tension equipment to pull my shoulder out of its comfort zone and to stretch it beyond its normal range of motion. It hurt, but it felt right.

By the first week of June, now that my shoulder was moving more freely, I was ready to drive again. I was still wearing T-shirts, sweatpants, and slip-on shoes for easy dressing. I drove down the mountain, paying very close attention to all the fundamentals and the goings-on around me.

I turned onto Broadway and headed north to get gas, figuring that this would be a good test for driving and negotiating the gas pump and credit card process. I pulled into the station and popped the gas cap. I fumbled with my wallet to get my credit card and slid it into the pump. The process went smoothly. I drove back up the mountain and proudly proclaimed myself a driver, capable of running errands in town.

Freedom! This opened up a world of options and did a lot for my psyche and confidence. I could now drive to the post office to mail our online store orders, cash checks at the bank, and even drive Barb the next time we went out for dinner. Up to this point I had shied away from playing tennis and socializing with friends, because I still felt so fragile and dependent. Regaining the ability to drive was a huge step for me, one I viewed as a major turning point.

I drove myself to therapy for the first time. I told Mary and Karen that I had started driving. Their reactions were the same: cautious at first, then pleased for me. I told Karen I was also ready to play tennis, so we worked on my shoulder with some tension and range of motion equipment. We also did some visual perception exercises. She pulled out a Superball and asked me to bounce it with my right hand and to catch it with my left, and vice versa, while standing still. Then I did the same thing as we walked down the hall. I could do it pretty well, but needed further practice.

After therapy I jumped in the car—or at least hopped—and called my friend Stuart to arrange a casual game of tennis for the next day; just some rallying and light running. That meant I had just that day to work on my ball toss for the serve, which was still a huge challenge. I got home and went to the side of the house to swing the racquet for a few minutes to loosen up the shoulder.

Barb, Ben, and I went out that evening for an early dinner, shortly after I began driving again. We arrived home and I positioned the car so I could back into the garage, as I'd done hundreds of times over the past two years. Barb's car was parked on the left side, so I used it as a guide from my side-view mirror, always keeping a good six inches from it. Ben and Barb were talking, and I was partially listening as I maneuvered the car. I felt a slight drag on the car and thought I must have sideswiped the garage frame on my left. Barb yelled, "Stop!" at the scraping noise, but I was slow to react and kept backing up. I got out of the car to find that I had actually sideswiped Barb's car, from wheel well to wheel well. She was livid, and I was immediately embarrassed and ashamed. The damage was relatively minor—just some scratched paint and surface creases—but even the smallest scratch translates into hundreds, if not thousands, of dollars.

The loss of money to repair the damage would be wrenching; but accepting my temporary lapse of concentration was even more painful. My hampered vision may have contributed to the accident, but in my mind the incident was more about my lack of respect for my condition. For months following this unfortunate occurrence, I had to relive this disaster in the form of warnings and reminders every time I backed into the garage. And I deserved them. But, just like the new neural pathways I had built for zipping my pants and closing my hand around a ball, I heeded Barb's warnings and remembered the catastrophe every time I parked the car, promising her that I would *never* make that mistake again. And I haven't.

Tennis – The Next Frontier (Eight Weeks)

I readied myself for the big day. I got my shorts and tennis shirt on with minimal hassle, but the socks took some time. I put on my tennis shoes for the first time and tried to tie them. Given my numb left hand, this presented a special challenge. I'd tried tying my laces a few times over the past two months, with no success, but thought today might be the day. After all, I could reach into the bottle of Plavix to take my daily pill, right?

Well, I had the skill to pinch the pill and get it to my mouth; but I could not feel it resting between my finger and thumb. This presented an interesting dynamic in the scope of recovery and weirdness. I had two issues with which to contend: my left hand was still too weak to master most small motor skills, such as tying laces and intertwining them, and my brain was still too mushy to visualize the process as I had once known it.

I could form two loops, the same way children do when they're first taught to tie their shoes. So there I sat with a loop in each hand. But there was a distinct disconnect between my hand and brain when I tried to recall the next step. I couldn't remember how I used to tie my shoes. I spent a few anxiety-filled minutes as I tried to envision the process. I moved my foot onto our bench and closer to my face. I made adjustments to my hand position to compensate for my inability to fully pronate and supinate—another challenge to overcome when tying laces. The anxiety was mounting, and I finally gave up and accepted that today would not be the day.

I drove down the mountain very carefully and made my way to the tennis club. My tennis partner, Stu, was hanging out with his dog, Blue. This was the first time he'd seen me since the stroke, so he asked how I was doing and we talked for a while. With some embarrassment and hesitation, I asked Stu to tie my shoes for me. I told him about all the strides I'd made and all the things I *could* do, but explained about my anxiety and inability to get past the loops. He's a sweet guy and gladly tied them for me, without too many wisecracks, even asking me if they were too tight.

We moved onto the court, and I pulled a racquet from my bag as he opened a can of balls. Stu handed me one ball to put in the pocket of my tennis shorts. Second dilemma of the day, after the shoe-tying fiasco: I couldn't get the ball into my pocket. Right-handed players put the ball in their left pocket, so they can keep their right hand on the racquet. The process of inserting a ball into my left pocket would need some examination.

I took a moment to review and break down the actual process, just as I'd done with so many other tasks I once took for granted. In the past I had held the ball in my left hand, and in one smooth motion I opened the fabric pocket and then slid in the ball: a natural and mindless process. To accomplish this "simple" task now, I would have to add an extra step to manually open the pocket before I put the ball in. The task was awkward and slow, but my friend waited patiently.

We took our sides and began rallying, as I assessed my capacity to run and hit the ball over the net. My swing was decent, and I could actually hit the ball. But I can't say that it was comfortable or natural, and when I ran it felt like my insides might fall out.

My vision and spatial awareness—and thus my relation to the ball—were not bad either, but I frequently found myself too close to the ball or too far behind it. Often I was overrunning shots. And my left side, which is my backhand side, was only marginally effective. My movements were stiff and jerky, and getting down to the ball in preparation for hitting a backhand was awkward and usually mistimed.

We stopped for some water, and Stu asked if I would like to play doubles with two women at the club, both of whom were decent players. I said sure, and we each took one as a partner. Stu took it upon himself to explain my condition, a role he seemed to enjoy and which he would perform each time we played doubles over the next few months. I didn't mind, nor did I feel self-conscious about it.

The girls warmed up, and we got down to playing. I explained that I would try to serve, but was not sure about my ability to toss the ball up. I knew that it would be good for me to try, and it would definitely loosen up my shoulder. They all agreed that my partner could take my service games if I couldn't serve.

We spun the racquet, and Stu was first to serve. I positioned myself behind the service box to receive. He looked straight at me and asked, with a straight face, "Should I take something off it because of your condition?"

I knew he'd made the comment in good humor, but it was also a slight dig, so I immediately did what guys do: I flipped him the bird, middle finger up. Third dilemma of the day: I was holding my racquet in my right hand, ready to receive serve, so I threw up my left hand, only to realize that I could not isolate the middle finger to deliver the message. I looked down at my hand to see all four fingers in a group, facing forward, looking unintelligible and far from the intended gesture. I looked at my hand, I looked at Stu, and we both broke up laughing. The girls didn't know me, and had no idea if I had a sense of humor about my condition, but they caught on and joined in.

It came time for me to serve. I went through the tossing motion, raising my left shoulder in a dry run without the ball. It was jerky and it hurt. After a short and somewhat frustrating struggle, I finally got the ball out of my left pocket. I stood at the baseline to bounce the ball a few times to get my rhythm, which is something I've always done. With the ball in my left hand, I tossed it up to serve.

In an unprecedented and totally bizarre sequence of events, I brought the racquet around and reached up to serve, only to realize that the ball was still stuck in my left claw. It had never released, and was still in my hand as I went to swing at it! I was speechless. In forty-five years of tennis, I'd never been so surprised or embarrassed.

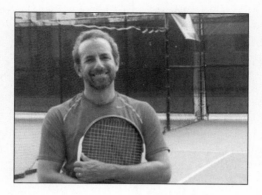

Stu and the girls saw this and cracked up. I was laughing so hard that it took me a full minute to recover my composure. I practiced the open and close motion a few times to get some neural messages to the hand, just like I had when I tried juggling for the first time.

Before the stroke I could play for hours, and I could run my ass off for a point and still recover in the twenty-five seconds before the next serve. Now I felt winded and a little fatigued, which in doubles had never been an issue, given that I only had to cover half the court. I'd have to see how this played out, but I thought it was most likely a result of being sedentary for so long.

Overall, though, I was satisfied with my first day out. I had played well, considering, and it broke the ice. I drove, I played tennis, I socialized, and I felt good about myself—a winner of a day all around.

In retrospect, that botched middle-finger gesture on the tennis court—along with Stu having to tie my tennis shoes—propelled me to the next level. One never knows how humiliation will turn the tide, and this was just one of those defining moments. I thought, "If I can't flip off a friend or tie my own shoes when I want, then just shoot me." I went home and really worked the Digi-Flex. I crumpled newspaper. I practiced with the Chinese balls. I did whatever I had to do to get control of my fingers. This fire in my belly proved that my will was strong enough to get me better. Within a week I could flip the bird when needed. Strangely enough, I had no one to flip off!

Another lesson: I remembered that it was important to think laterally during rehabilitation. This meant that if better finger control helped flip the bird, then it would probably help me improve in other troubled or deficient areas. Considering this, I grabbed my guitar off the stand and played a few notes, and then the infamous D-chord. I saw some improvement in each area. I could just about form the chord, but I could tell that something else was off. Like the day I struggled to put the laptop into the docking station before finally realizing that it was missing the connection by an inch, I had been playing the chord on the wrong fret—about an inch off.

Chapter 15

TRAVELING

B arb and I had planned a trip to San Diego to visit our son
Bryan and his girlfriend, Kim, before I had my stroke. We
decided we would go ahead with the visit, despite my limitations. The reality of traveling finally hit me. I felt apprehensive
about every aspect of the process—even getting my shoes off
and on at the airport security gate. I was concerned about my
energy level and worried that I wouldn't be able to get my
much-needed afternoon naps. But I was still excited. More
than anything, I looked at this trip as a week of relaxation
and rejuvenation, away from my therapy, the command center, and my den. I still intended to do my therapy, so I packed
the Chinese balls, the Digi-Flex, a set of drumsticks, and my
Thera-band, along with my tennis racquet and dancing shoes.
I'd grown quite attached to my guitar and considered it to be
one of the best forms of therapy. I did some research on the
Internet and found a music shop in Encinitas where I could
rent one.

The drive to Denver International Airport was the first
time I'd taken the wheel on a highway, and driving at higher
speeds proved to be a bit challenging. I felt tentative, but
good. Because of my left field vision cut, I felt a little distant
and removed from the road, and I worked extra hard to stay
in my lane. I successfully navigated the roads leading into the
airport parking lots and was totally surprised when I got pulled
over for speeding. Barb and I were deep in conversation, and
my mind was not on the speedometer. I begged for leniency,
but still got a $130 ticket and two points on my license.

We landed in San Diego, rented a car, and hit the highway north to Encinitas. I felt like a kid on his first trip to the beach. I smelled the ocean air and basked in the sunshine with all the windows open.

Our old friends from Ann Arbor, Tom and Carol, had moved to Del Mar, and we had visited them once before my stroke. Tom had suffered a bizarre back injury, which led to major surgery that left him with serious paralysis from the waist down. One day he was playing golf with his buddies, and the next day he was bedridden with severe back pain and some paralysis. The day after that he was in surgery and facing an uphill battle to regain his ability to walk.

We called Tom and Carol to say that we were in Encinitas and set a dinner date for Thursday night in Del Mar, at a seafood restaurant fifty yards from the crashing surf. We met there and found them at the bar. Tom was in a wheelchair, which was a strange sight. Carol grabbed his drink as Tom wheeled himself over to our table. We talked for hours about his injury, his daily therapy, and the very long, slow road to what we all hoped would be complete recovery.

The last time we visited I was still healing from my dislocated shoulder, but was moving a hell of a lot better than he was. We broke the news about my stroke and my own paralysis, then shared war stories about the hospital, physical therapy, and such. We talked at length about his daily therapy and the challenges he was facing trying to learn to walk without the aid of a walker or crutches. Most of his legs and both of his feet were still numb, with pretty severe nerve damage. His feet were also bent and pronated, which made it impossible for him to set his feet flat on the ground. Because of this, he dragged more than he walked, even with the use of his aids.

I sensed that he was very frustrated and dissatisfied with his slow improvement and was becoming depressed and defeated. I also sensed that most of his therapy was being done at the rehab hospital, with supervision. He went to rehab most days, for two or three hours, but to really improve he would have to work at it diligently at home every day, without a therapist to egg him on. Carol worked full-time and was already losing precious hours running him to doctors and therapy.

Tom and I go way back, so I couldn't help thinking that smoking a little pot might do him a lot of good, given his situation, the long road ahead—and the fact that medical marijuana was legal in California. I wouldn't have even brought it up if he weren't so beaten and depressed. He was literally trapped inside his body. I knew how he felt. I told him about what smoking did for me and regaled him with the details of my first experience under the influence, when I tried to juggle. He smiled, but I could see his mind racing. We had a fine time with our friends, and it was great to connect. We said our goodbyes and drove back to Encinitas.

I got up early, as usual, while Barb slept in. I loved the early morning walks on the beach, with the surf lapping up against my ankles. It became a daily routine for me to walk a few miles, maybe sit and watch and reflect for a while, followed by a heart-pounding race back up the stairs to street level.

Along with the tennis I'd been playing, this was the first exercise I'd done at sea level, and I found it so much easier than the workouts I'd been doing in Boulder, at 5,500 feet elevation.

After my walk and stair-running, I had some time to kill before Barb got up, so I devoted some quality time to the tying of my shoes. I'd had enough of flip-flops and slip-on shoes, even though I was at the beach and could have gotten away with them for the rest of the week.

I sat on the floor staring at my tennis shoes. I focused on the laces and mentally tried to tie them while the shoes sat in front of me, off my feet. The process was kind of like trying to tie someone else's necktie, and just as confusing to coordinate.

I put the shoes on and lifted my left foot onto the coffee table. I made the first tie and then formed a bow on the right, which was always the easiest part. The next part was the one that had confounded me in previous attempts. In the past, I had the right bow formed, wrapped the lace over the bow to do the left side, but then got lost. This time I got the bow ready and I wrapped the lace over the bow and around my right thumb. All I had to do was get the lace through the bow and I would be done.

This time around I finally understood the angle and the goal with a renewed clarity. The lace went through without a hitch, but I couldn't articulate the final step with my left forefinger, so I pushed the lace through with my right and: ta-da! I had tied my shoe.

I methodically repeated the process five times to forge the new neural pathway and to get the movement into my muscle memory.

I ran into the bedroom and woke Barb with a celebratory kiss.

"I tied my shoe! I tied my shoe!"

I found time each day to play guitar and work out with the Digi-Flex and Chinese balls. I even sneaked in a few naps. But I connected most with the dancing at night. When I danced, I moved my entire body in coordinated, rhythmic ways that straight therapy could not provide. Stroke, in my case, had hit my whole body, even though the worst physical damage occurred in my left shoulder, arm, and hand. My body went from being flexible and responsive to being stiff and foreign, with a bunch of disconnected limbs. Dancing, with its unstructured movement and freedom, was what I needed to regain my physical sense of self. That night, in celebration, I wore laced shoes to dance in.

At the bar I drank a beer and began moving my body in my seat. When I stepped onto the dance floor, I felt stiff and stupid. I could hear and feel the beat, but my body was a step or two slow and a bit out of sync. When the song ended I ordered another beer and a shot, which changed my whole attitude. I'd been too much in my head and couldn't escape the confines of my body.

I listened to the music, I moved my limbs, and I got into it. Barb and I danced until 1 AM, and it was, bar none, the best thing I could have done for my body and mind. We danced most nights for the whole vacation.

Chapter 16

THE NEXT LEVEL

Another Epiphany (June 15, 2008)

At the bar, I noticed something revealing about my hands and arms. We were sitting on a stool, snuggled up close to the edge of the bar. I had an empty Heineken bottle in my left hand, holding it as if I were drinking it. I turned my wrist to the left as far as I could to see if I could touch the bottle-neck to the top of the bar. I could not. In fact, it was three inches from touching. I turned my wrist to the right and tried it in that direction, with the same result. We thought that if I could touch the bottle to the bar while Barb pushed it down, it would stretch my wrist or ligaments and facilitate a better range of motion. We repeated this a few times, thinking we might be on to something.

The repetition and force of Barb's hand did not make a difference, but it did help us come to the conclusion that my inability to pronate, and thus touch the bar top, was not a wrist or hand issue as much as it was a shoulder issue. I decided at that moment to begin a new exercise on my own as soon as we got home.

After unpacking and settling back in, I tested my theory. I lay on my back on the rug in the den and spread my arms out to the sides. Then, keeping the backs of my arms extended and pressed to the floor with my palms up, I slowly swept them above my head, as if I were making a snow angel. The right arm went up to the twelve o'clock position smoothly, with no pain. I felt a little stretch, but it was totally within my comfort zone. But on the left side I had to stop halfway up because the pain was so intense. I also noticed that, while my right elbow and arm remained on the rug all the way up to my ear, my left would not. By the time my left arm reached halfway, my elbow was three inches above the rug.

I sat up and marveled at this revelation. I knew immediately what I had to do. I also knew it would take a long time and it would hurt like shit. There would be no instant gratification on this one.

I decided to commit ten minutes a day for two weeks to extreme stretching, regardless of the pain, until my left arm could touch my left ear without lifting my elbow or arm off the rug. If after two weeks it didn't improve, then I would see the doctor and get an MRI. I really had to follow my gut here. It was only pain, and I could handle pain. It would be much more painful to live with a frozen shoulder and have to compromise my lifestyle.

The next morning I went straight to the den to start my stretching routine. I warmed up the arm and shoulder, and then got into the proper position on my back. I brought both arms up toward my ears, trying to match the left to the movement and flexibility of my right. I used my right arm to gently bring the left one along. It hurt worse than anything I'd experienced before; enough to bring tears to my eyes. I moved the left arm closer and closer to my ear, inch by inch, nudging it along with my right. Each inch was literal agony, but I still felt I was doing the right thing. I repeated the exercise at night before bed.

I woke up the next morning with a dull, deep pain in my left shoulder. I massaged in some sports cream to help with the discomfort and then got into position to repeat the stretching process from the day before. I did this twice a day for the next two weeks.

Midweek, I went to PT for what was hopefully going to be my last regularly scheduled therapy session. I shared my theory about the scar tissue with Karen and then showed her my new routine. She kind of sighed—mostly out of concern, I thought—and then she gently warned me about my approach.

"You could hurt yourself; you could pull something. Pain is not always necessary in order to heal."

I heard her and I thanked her, but told her again that it felt right to me, and that I intended to see the next week-and-a-half through on my own. I would keep her posted.

Still Working It (Almost Ten Weeks)

I had definitely moved on to the next level. I did the dishes every night after dinner. Doing the glasses had gotten easier as my hand became more responsive, but I really had to concentrate to hold onto the slick, soapy surface. I could handle larger items better. Small items such as spoons, forks, and knives still stumped me. For instance, I couldn't yet feel the single Plavix that I took each morning. Turning the pages of a magazine or book and handling money were still very slow going.

At the end of the two weeks of painful and often tearful stretching, my shoulder was feeling better. I had a greatly improved range of motion, with tolerable pain and discomfort. This translated into a much better tennis ball toss and much more power on my serve. When driving I was able to turn the steering wheel freely, and I could fasten the seatbelt without wincing. Things were looking up.

During the last three days of my shoulder work, with assistance from my right arm, I began pulling and extending my left arm above my head and against my left ear. It felt like I was pulling the arm out of the socket, but it was definitely helping. I added this exercise to my morning stretches and continued working it every day, without fail. I found this shoulder rehabilitation an amazing experience, one I will always appreciate and will never forget—not only because it worked, but because it proved to me something I believe we all know, deep inside: Our bodies will tell us what they need to heal, if we can only listen.

I got back to my tennis regimen of playing two to three times a week, but my respiratory problem was still an issue, especially when playing singles. To address this condition, and in an effort to improve it, I made my first after-stroke attempt at hiking Mount Sanitas, a local Boulder mountain just two minutes from downtown. I had done this hike ten times, often running up segments when spurts of energy propelled me. This two-hour hike took me up 1,500 feet. The hike was steeper than it was technically challenging, so it would make a good training ground and an excellent barometer by which to judge my growing strength and stamina.

I set out on a beautiful, hot, sunny June day. I had started slowly on the flats at the bottom, working my way up to the steeper stuff, when my cell phone rang. It was my friend Susan, asking if I was coming to play tennis, as I was already ten minutes late! I was so damned embarrassed to have spaced this out. I had made an entry in my datebook and even kept her email in my inbox, so I would see it each time I was at the computer. I'd never missed a tennis date in my whole life. I lived for tennis, and it was always at the top of my list. I apologized twice and even offered to come right away, but she had to leave.

This was a huge wakeup call for me. I'd actually looked at my datebook just before I left for Sanitas and had completely glazed over it, even though—as I discovered when I got home—the appointment was written in red ink.

I realized this was both a visual and a cognitive issue. But I berated myself over and over during the hike and was initially too embarrassed to mention the event to Barb. I was so very disappointed in myself. I knew that I was not fully healed, but I'd sure felt like I was getting there. My bubble of denial was once again popped.

I did not do well on the hike. My footing was good and my balance was better than it had been a month ago, but I got too winded to make it to the top, which I had done successfully and energetically every previous time.

I did a lot of thinking about my life and my goals during the hike. The tennis calamity weighed heavily on me, and I couldn't get it off my mind. I knew my therapists had told me to be patient and to accept these mishaps graciously, but I had really failed. I became nervous and paranoid about missing calls and meetings. From that point on, I color-coded all the entries in my datebook and used yellow highlighter to emphasize important meetings. I also made additional notes on sticky pads and posted them in strategic places: in my command center; at the top of the stairs; on the dashboard of my car.

There's a tendency during recovery to accept less-than-perfect performance when one sees improvement, which then causes the injured person to slow down and even curtail the work they do at home. I had discovered myself to be somewhat guilty of this, so I learned a valuable lesson that day: "Better" is not necessarily "all better."

I know a guy who suffered a bad leg injury from skiing that required extensive surgery. He completed minimal physical therapy before he stopped attending sessions. As a result of this decision, he now walks with a severe limp. Lesson: We owe our body and brain the most complete recovery possible, so do not give up until you are as close to "normal" as possible—and don't go soft on this issue, because you will have to live with your decision for the rest of your hopefully long life.

Now that I could think and comprehend a bit more clearly, I wanted answers to a number of questions about my stroke; the subsequent procedure in which they put the stent into my carotid artery; and my quality of life in the years to come.

I questioned my doctors about the stent and my ability to play sports going forward. Dr. Zacharias and Dr. Mao both said that I should be able to ski, body surf, and partake in most sports without concern. However, I should be aware that a hit or shock to my neck could bend, fracture, or break the stent, which may not be fatal, but would require immediate medical help. I should stay away from wrestling and "neck locks"— which should not be too hard at my age—and be careful when doing any contact sports or sports that involve impact.

"So far, so good," I had to concede. I just wouldn't take up boxing.

When I went in for the CT angio as planned, I was not nearly as uncomfortable and afraid of the hospital environment as I had been before the stroke and during my five-day stay. But it was hard to be back in the hospital with an IV in my arm. I felt hopeful, yet a little fearful about the results. I'd been told that if the test results were all good, I might be taken off Plavix, so there was an additional plus to getting a clean bill of health.

I worried for the three days it took to get the results of the CT scan, but everything looked fine. A CT angiogram is not completely conclusive, because there's only so much they can see from the test. Dr. Zacharias was hesitant about taking me off Plavix just yet, but did ultimately give his seal of approval. I would, however, be taking 81 milligrams of aspirin every day. I understand that this is common procedure with stroke and heart attack victims, but the thought of taking aspirin every day, or taking anything for the rest of my life other than vitamins, felt weird, controlling, and invasive. I joked that at least I would probably never get another headache!

I could feel a distinct difference in my body and respiratory system within two weeks of getting off the Plavix. I noticed it first in my tennis and rollerblading. Months later I hiked up Mount Sanitas again and was able to make the summit, without the stress and the huffing and puffing. I also experienced better concentration and took fewer naps in the coming months.

Chapter 17

WIMBLEDON

Two Months and Three Weeks

I was hoping to feel well enough to go to Wimbledon, the oldest and most elite tennis tournament in the world, and the only Grand Slam event that's played on grass. I had never been to England. Wimbledon is just one of the major tournaments won by my tennis hero, Rod Laver—on his way to an unprecedented two Grand Slams (all four major titles in one year)—and my other tennis hero, John Newcombe, both of whom had suffered strokes in the past decade. ("Newk" wrote the foreword to this book.)

Even though I had made the San Diego trip and had done reasonably well, this was a nine-hour flight, and I would definitely miss all my nap time while away. Plus, I would be traveling all by myself. But the trip would be amazing: the tennis, the cultural experience, the rest and relaxation, the change of environment. After three months of therapy and doctors, I was psyched to go.

I would be meeting up with Gary Addie while I was in London. Gary was my oldest and closest friend, a tennis teaching pro, and a beautiful player in his own right. His mom won Wimbledon in 1946, which was the only year she played it because of the war. For you tennis buffs, her name is Pauline Betz, and she also scooped up four U.S. championships between 1942 and 1946. As a past Wimbledon champion, Pauline has an option to buy premier seats every year. As luck would have it, Gary asked me again this year, shortly after my stroke. I accepted with gratitude. Of course, with the U.S. dollar devalued at approximately half, it would be an expensive trip. Still . . . Wimbledon!

We were scheduled to be there for seven days, with six fantastic days of tennis. This promised to be very therapeutic, because all I had to do was sit on my ass for eight hours a day and watch the best tennis players in the world compete for the foremost title in the sport.

Here we were, as the beneficiaries of Pauline's tickets, with two Court One seats and two Centre Court seats. I felt like royalty. Outside the gates of Wimbledon, people of all ages waited patiently in anticipation of entering the land of grass and refinement. They started showing up as early as 6 AM to queue for grounds passes, the ones that would entitle them to walk around the club and see matches on the outside courts. Unlike the queues in America, these people stand in an orderly line and chat. You will not see Brits queuing at Wimbledon with coolers of beer, turning rowdy and unruly.

We had the honor and good fortune to actually play on grass courts toward the middle of our stay. Gary's very kind and sweet friends, Mark and Elizabeth, took us to the Hurlingham Club, a venerable English establishment founded in 1869. I wasn't feeling my best, and I moved a bit slowly on the court, but it was still a dream come true: my very heartfelt thanks to Mark and Elizabeth for their invitation and gracious manner.

Getting out of our hotel room each morning in time for the matches became a comedy of errors. Each night when we returned to the hotel from a late dinner, I would undress and line up all of my possessions from the day at the matches. This way, most of what I needed for the next day would be easy to find each morning. Without this continuity and order, it would have taken me forever to get out the door. Even with this planned and apparent order, I still felt anxious and vulnerable when trying to pack my pockets for the day.

In the movie *It's a Wonderful Life* with James Stewart and Donna Reed, and a cast of other greats, there's a character named Clarence who plays the guardian angel who comes down from heaven to look after George Bailey. Clarence explains that there's a jingle of bells every time an angel gets its wings. I had this image in my mind every time I did something "strokelike," such as misplacing my pass for the Tube, spacing something out, or just standing in a daze. I would hear a *rrring* in my head, like a high-pitched bell. I told Gary about this, and from then on, whenever I did something that was clearly a result of my stroke I would lift my right index finger, point it toward the sky, and make an audible *rrring* sound. It became a euphemism for my condition, and it saved me from having to explain myself every time. While it became a running joke for the remainder of the trip, in reality it was a poignant way of recognizing my condition without making a big deal of it.

Thursday morning, which was the fourth day of our trip, we got up early to rollerblade before the matches. Gary and I walked through the lobby and sat down on a curb to the right of the hotel entrance to put on our blades. Gary just carried his skates and pads in his hands, wearing only socks on his feet. I wore my Nike flip-flops and carried my boot bag because I wasn't good at keeping track of all the various parts. When I was done, almost five minutes after Gary, I packed up the boot bag and gave it to the concierge, who graciously offered to put it behind his desk while we skated. I returned to the curb to begin blading and realized that I had inadvertently left one of my flip-flops out of the bag. Gee, what a surprise: *rrring*!

I didn't want to make an issue of it, or inconvenience the concierge, so I looked around for a place to stash the flip-flop till we got back. There was a forty-foot row of hedges lining the front left side of the hotel, so I discretely stashed the flip-flop in an opening in the shrub, neatly positioned so no one could see it.

The streets of Camden were a bit bumpy, which doesn't make for the best rollerblading, but the views of the villages and townships, with their stone and brick row houses and palatial estates, were quaint and glorious. It's a damn good thing I had skated once in Boulder before dragging my blades to London, because it gave me enough confidence to meet the challenges of a new area, with new terrain and unfamiliar driving patterns: I looked both ways twice before crossing these roads because the cars drive on the "wrong" side of the road.

We returned from a rousing skate and sat back down on the curb in front of the hotel to take off our gear. We were on an adrenaline high from the skate and feeling a bit giddy about the tennis matches ahead of us. I reached into the hedge to retrieve my flip-flop but could not find it. I looked at Gary, figuring I had spaced it out and was looking in the wrong place. At that exact moment, a very proper British employee of the hotel stuck his head out of the glass door and said, in the best "butler" English lilt, "Are you looking for yore shyoo?"

I started laughing because it was just so goddamn weird. Though stunned, I eventually spit out, "Yes, I am!"

· He eyed me without smiling and said, "The concierge has it."

I apologized for the obvious faux pas as casually as I could, but felt very embarrassed.

He assured me it was "No problem atoll, sir."

I looked at Gary and spun my right finger to the sky, then skulked into the lobby to retrieve my flip-flop.

The concierge, recognizing me, said rather loudly, "Are you looking for yore shyoo?"

I stammered out a self-conscious, "Yes, I am" and then

mumbled, "Was there an email or a bulletin sent out to the whole hotel?"

He smiled very politely and handed me my boot bag and flip-flop. The latter he held forth gingerly, as if it had been retrieved from a barnyard.

One of the guys in our group, another Steve, had quite a lot to say about my condition. I had shared the stories of my spacey experiences, my forgetfulness, and my anxiety when gathering my possessions each morning. Steve was sixty-two, nine years older than me. He has an MBA and is an accomplished businessman with a lot on his plate. Steve said that what I was describing is actually his life, and he's never had a stroke! He has to write down everything, from phone numbers to appointments, and didn't think my mental condition was that unusual. That admission didn't make me feel all that good about my future.

Chapter 18

GETTING BACK TO IT!

By the fifth month following the stroke, I had regained almost full use of my left shoulder, though I still suffered regular bouts of tingling and numbness. Using a fork was still a challenge. I normally hold it with my right hand to eat, which was fine, but when I switched it to the left so I could hold the knife in my right hand to cut my food, I could not hold the fork with the tines facing forward. The fork would naturally fall sideways and continue to slip from my hand. So I repositioned it, patiently. And often. Call it stubbornness, vanity, or ego, but I felt I had graduated from the "fat fork" when I left the hospital, and I was not going back.

The numbness in my left hand had diminished, but I still fumbled when turning the pages of a magazine or newspaper and when handling paper money, because three of my fingers seemed to have a mind of their own. Typing was also a fiasco, slow and laborious at times. I often hit the Caps Lock key on the keyboard with my spastic left-hand fingers, SO THE REST OF THE SENTENCE LOOKED LIKE THIS. Typing this book was an incredible challenge and at times very frustrating, as I was unable to type as fast as I can think (even though I don't think as fast as I once did!).

I realized that my left hand became very fatigued by repetitive motions and made a mental note to devise an exercise to strengthen that problem.

Here's my point: Experiment. Design your own exercises and run them by your physical therapist to make sure they are suited to your deficits and abilities. Each task you master may yield unexpected benefits in some other area—which in turn can lead to greater opportunities for improvement.

I noticed a number of deficits in my day-to-day life during the writing of this book; I wanted to make sure I was not slipping backwards, so I went to see Karen at PT to get a checkup. She took one look at my wandering eyes and knew that I still had work to do. She could see my peripheral vision waning and wasted no time telling me. I was so happy to be back in the mainstream that I had neglected my eye exercises. My thinking processes were still slowed, particularly if they involved reading or specific verbal instruction. With each mishap or hiccup comes the chance to build a new neural pathway to retrain my mind and body. Each time I had a finger-in-the-air-moment, I would make a point of repeatedly performing the process I needed to learn until it was cemented in.

NIA

Besides tennis, my exercises of choice are Neuromuscular Integrative Action (NIA) and Soul Sweat. NIA mixes movement, dance, balance, and Tae Kwon Do, all set to music, so there's a good amount of physicality to it—and a great deal of fun. I believe that classic NIA may be the best all-around physical therapy a stroke victim can do, assuming that they're capable of expressing the required range of motion. I take NIA classes twice a week.

NIA serves a mixed bag of people of various ages and skill levels. In most classes, the teacher will openly tell you to do the step at whatever level is comfortable and will demonstrate, saying, "Level One can do it this way, Level Two can do it this way," and so on. NIA classes may not be the place for people who cannot move their body, or who need individual attention. However, the classes can be the perfect place to move the body in rhythmic motion and to judge improvement, week by week. Just as you would when learning anything new, it's essential to stay patient with yourself and give it some time. It does take a certain level of commitment to improve.

For many months after the stroke I found NIA both challenging and humbling. I had tremendous problems following the steps and mastering direction—often going left when I should be going right and vice versa. My mistakes were embarrassing, but my progress has been worth it; I could see my improvement as the months went by. The movements taxed my cognitive and physical abilities, which clearly identified my deficits. For example, I felt a profound imbalance between my left and right arms and hands when kicking, jabbing and punching. I vowed to practice these movements until I felt a better, more natural balance.

NIA classes are available throughout most of the United States. Check out www.nianow.com for information and studio locations. And don't be shy about explaining your situation or limitations, as NIA teachers are trained to teach all body types and most body conditions, from pregnant women to people in recovery to accomplished athletes.

Even if you've never danced before, now would be the time to start. Dancing has become the best physical therapy I can do for my body and mind. The physical demands are great and it takes a lot of endurance, but the reliance on spatial awareness and the need to combine steps really work both my left and right brain functions. Now, if I can only learn to do it all on beat! The main thing is just to move your body to music. Music has remarkable powers to stimulate the brain. The type of dance or movement is less important than the movement itself. Whatever rocks your boat: salsa, swing, African, Jazzercise, ballroom; anything that takes you out of the particular space that is holding you back, either mentally or physically.

Creating Your Own Therapy Sessions (Six Months)

I've found that therapy comes in many shapes and guises. You can take what you've learned from therapy and modify it to fit your needs as you progress, or you can create your own therapies. Once you can read your body and understand what a specific therapy does for it, you can use just about anything to customize a therapy and incorporate it into your routine. There's also a value in discovering something on your own that feeds a need and works for you. Of course, always be sure to run these by your doctor or physical therapist to make sure you're not doing more harm than good.

I have tools and toys in my wicker basket in the den, but sometimes I grow bored, or I'm on the go without them. I was out one evening killing time at a restaurant and was absent-mindedly rolling my cell phone over and over in my right hand—from the flat part to the edge and over to the flat part again, rolling it from my palm to my fingertips, much like the Chinese balls. It was a smooth motion, it had rhythm, and I liked the feel. I immediately tried it in my left hand and found it hard to do and not as rhythmic—an obvious deficiency. I am still committed to making my left hand as capable as my right, so this turned out to be an appealing discovery and a routine I could do anywhere.

(Be sure to check out the list of other "home" therapies in the section titled Exercises for Therapy at the end of this book.)

Another very good therapy, which many guys in my age group might never discover, is folding laundry. My wife does most of the folding in our house, even though I am a clothing-care expert. As it happened, Barb was out of town for four days, so I did a load of socks, shirts, and underwear.

Early on in my rehabilitation, I would take off a pair of pants at night and try to re-hang them. I would lay the pants on the bed, fold one leg over the other, and try to match the side seams. I could not fold them, or even envision the process. After a full minute or so of fumbling, and sensing that I was done trying, Barb would take them from me and finish the job. It looked a lot easier than it was.

This time, during Barb's absence, I found folding laundry to be excellent therapy. Folding clothing, depending on how anal you are (or your wife is), requires dexterity and patience to line up seams and smooth out wrinkles. I can't say that I was such a stickler for doing things that came hard to me before my stroke, but now, every time I find another deficiency I celebrate it and try to improve.

Tell Others What You Need

Six months after my stroke, I had made so much physical improvement that Barb sometimes overestimated my mental condition and expected too much of me. I appreciated her confidence, but I still had a long way to go. She teased me occasionally, which is fine because we both have to keep a sense of humor, but she needed to recognize that I was still not all there.

After thirty years of marriage, and going through the stroke together, Barb and I are almost one person. Yet, as close as we are—and as intuitive as she is—there's just no way that she—or anybody else—could fully understand the fog inside my head. Coming back from a stroke and regaining "normal" brain functions is much like physical rehabilitation, but people cannot see inside the brain the way they can see physical recovery as it unfolds. I told Barb that she needed to be totally blunt with me; this kind of open, honest communication is essential to a successful recovery.

Sports: Moving Forward

I struggled with the thought of skiing again. It's late August and colder than usual; snow had fallen in the mountains at ten thousand feet and above. The tallest peaks, visible from Boulder, had been snowcapped all summer, so skiing was never really off my mind. But neither was what happened the last time I went skiing. Soon I would be ready, but not yet.

In October, almost eight months after the stroke, Barb and I drove to Moab, Utah, for some hiking and kayaking. This was my first long drive since the stroke, and it was a good test of my ability to stay focused for six hours at a time.

We entered the park and hiked a few miles, up and around boulders and ledges, when we came to a long path at the top of a ridge. The ridge top was maybe eight feet wide and reasonably flat, with a drop-off of forty feet on one side and two hundred feet on the other. People of all ages were walking this path to sit on the edge of the precipice, so we followed.

Twenty feet along the path, I had to stop in my tracks. Saying that I had a strong feeling of imbalance would be an understatement; I was stricken and unable to continue. In all my years of hiking, I'd never experienced this fear and uncertainty. I could not move. Just standing on the path felt overwhelming. I actually had to sit my ass down on the rock path to reduce my anxiety.

I told Barb what I was feeling and encouraged her to continue on if she was interested. She chose to stay back, urging me to listen to my mind and body. We sat on the ledge of a large boulder and talked about it while hikers ventured down the path.

I used to literally *run* over terrain like this, picking and choosing which rock to bounce off of like a mountain goat. A rush of inadequacy washed over me, and I felt deeply confused. We sat for twenty minutes and then turned around and followed trails to flat terrain that led to some other arches.

The final descent took us over some uneven rocks and small boulders, with very little vertical drop on either side. But I was so shaken by my earlier fear that even this terrain scared me. My trail-running shoes felt as if they had no grip, even though they did. I crouched closer to the surface to lower my center of gravity, and for the rockier sections I actually had to crawl down on my butt. A year after my stroke, I still haven't gotten over this newfound fear and vertigo. I will have to face these demons again as I get better in the months and years to come.

Barb and I made another trip to Pacific Beach to visit Bryan. We arranged to have Ben fly out as well, so we could all be together for the first time since my stroke. We set up a tennis match for the next morning, followed by a bodysurfing session in the ocean.

In a letter Bryan wrote to me shortly after my stroke, he'd said:

"As far as I'm concerned, you are back to the same person I have grown up with my whole life. You are stroke-proof, if not bulletproof, and I will *kick your sorry ass in tennis* with no remorse the next time we meet!"

I never forgot this playful threat, and used it as inspiration during my recovery. Pacific Beach was the perfect opportunity to take his challenge head-on! I watched Bryan and Ben go at each other until it was my turn to play against each son, one-on-one. I won both of my matches, playing much more sure-footedly than the last time we visited Bryan! Unfortunately, Bryan twisted an ankle before we could settle our friendly feud, so we had to cut it short and head for the beach.

(I'm glad to report that on our latest visit with Bryan in March of 2009, eleven months after my stroke, he did exact some retribution by winning the first two games of 21 with a slew of hard, powerful forehands and backhands. In the next three games, I regained my composure and ultimately won the best of five!)

Ben ran into the waves, and I walked out slowly as I acclimated to the water. We stood next to each other in waist-deep surf, waiting for the right wave to ride. I picked a small one to start, caught it exactly right, and rode that baby in. The exhilaration and joy came rushing back to me! I kept my extended arms very tight against my neck and ears to protect my neck and carotid artery, but I still felt vulnerable and slightly fearful. I will have to deal with this as I move forward.

Cognition

Healing comes in different forms, and the *meaning* of healing changes with each slice of time. At first it seemed that my mind and my body were healing at the same speed. After a few months, however, it seemed that my cognitive development was proceeding more slowly than my physical development. Even with my spastic left hand, lifeless fingers, and numb arm, my body still basically functioned. When most of the body works as it should, the mind gets false signs and it takes a little siesta. By the six-month mark, as I accepted my body and got back to routine physical exercise, my mind started to show cracks and weaknesses. My mental improvement seemed to have taken a backseat to my physical recovery.

I now believe that my mind will take years to catch up. Here's a case in point: I met a friend for tennis and pulled my tennis bag out of the trunk of my car. I left my wallet on the floor of the trunk in place of the tennis bag, figuring I would reclaim the wallet when I put the bag back in the trunk after tennis. I did put the bag back in the same place, but did not even think about the wallet or retrieving it. That night I dressed for a dinner date downtown and could not find my wallet. I looked in my pants, in my tennis shorts, on the hall table where I usually put it, and methodically searched my mind as I retraced my steps, but finally gave up in frustration and confusion. It was dark outside, so I took a flashlight from the kitchen to look on the tennis court as a last resort. On the way to dinner, I had a flash and searched to the left of my tennis bag in the trunk, and the wallet was still there. But look at the stress and hassle I had to endure!

As I've said before, many "normal" fifty-somethings have memory issues, and Barb is quick to add that even before the stroke I was one of the worst offenders when it came to misplacing my wallet—but I am now ten times worse. These recent mishaps come from a different, deeper place, and are not just the result of being fifty-three and spacey. These occurrences are huge disconnects that have tested my recall, my ability to reason, and my fragile short-term memory.

I intend to work harder to develop processes to address these deficiencies. Yes, it could take years for my Humpty-Dumpty brain to put all its pieces back together again—but given my experience and the success of my therapeutic experiments, I have no doubt that I'll get there.

And I know that you can too.

The brain is plastic; it changes and grows as we do, and it continues to change throughout our lifetime. So even though different folks have different strokes, one thing remains a constant: Recovering from a stroke is a creative endeavor. It requires patience, determination, and stamina. But most of all, we can all benefit from listening to the intuitive leaps that tell *us* what will work best for us on *our* road to recovery. And sometimes we may even find we're functioning better than we did before!

I may not think as quickly or recall as easily where I left my wallet. But there's a lot to be said for an increase in compassion, a deeper understanding of the mysterious ways of the mind and body, and an unending gratitude for every day of my life.

EPILOGUE

Changes Come in the Strangest Packages (One Year)

In the space of twelve months, I went from the depths of despair to new heights of personal discovery. I couldn't put two thoughts together, and I struggled with basic math and reading. In the fog of those early days I did a lot of thinking; like a young child who listens and observes, taking it all in, but does not yet speak. When he does, though, he speaks volumes.

Most people tend to be set in their ways when they reach fifty, and changes do not come easily. But it's almost impossible to go through a major upheaval like a stroke and not be changed. Most stroke survivors will surely agree.

So here's where I've landed a year after my stroke:

First of all, I do not consider myself a victim. I consider myself to be incredibly lucky. If you had asked me a year ago to predict how I would feel if I ever had a stroke, I would have been horrified even to imagine it. Yet this has been the most illuminating year of my life. I can honestly say that I feel fortunate to have experienced both the good *and* the bad of the last twelve months.

As we get older, most of us reflect on our passage through this world: childhood, school, work, family. We also examine our mortality. We might think about our value as a human being, and whether or not we've done all we could do and been all we could be. We might have regrets and wish we had done some things differently in our lives, or in our children's lives. There's so much to consider when you feel your own mortality acutely at such a young age—and these, days fifty-three is young.

In my case, I thought that I'd lived a good life, with few doubts and few regrets. But after having a stroke, and having to relearn the fundamentals that I'd taken for granted most of my life, I've changed my tune on many levels; from the way I misunderstood and related to disabled and elderly people, to the way I raced through my days, to the raising of my children. No, I have not been suddenly "born again," per se. My experience has been much more gradual and grounded than that. I felt things changing in me after the stroke, but I caught only glimpses that I could not yet touch or articulate. I sensed that all would be revealed in time. As it turns out, insights and discoveries come to you in the strangest ways.

During the summer, Boulder throws a weekly concert on its pedestrian mall. I was sitting with Barb at one of these—listening to a fantastic Beatles tribute band—when I got up to buy a bottle of water. It had one of those newfangled tab tops that have always confused me, even before the stroke: the top has a small plastic rip tab that has to be released before the top can be flipped open. I've always hated them, and I know I'm not the only one.

Soon I was embroiled in a personal battle of wits. I wanted to ask the college kid behind the counter for help, or take a pair of pliers to demolish the tab top, but instead decided then and there that I would face and defeat my demons. Just a showdown between me and this goddamn bottle. I studied it from all angles, played with the tab, twisted the cap, which did not budge, and tried to break the seal and flip the top.

At that exact moment, I had an epiphany; a true revelation. Since the stroke, I'd had to relearn almost every task. Staring at the water bottle, lost in my own little world, I realized that I am no longer satisfied with the status quo. Everything *had* changed. The water bottle was just the messenger.

Every task I learned after the stroke took patience, repetition, will, and fortitude. The simplest things took all of me. I had to break down every aspect of every task. Before the stroke, I gave up too easily. I accepted defeat too easily and, on some level, took the easy way out too often, which made me weaker and less capable. Even though I grew to become an accomplished businessperson, writer, and parent, I could now see—with incredible clarity—that I was a different person, and I would never be satisfied with the way things were before.

With this revelation, I felt ecstatic and otherworldly. I started racing through the things I'd relearned, one by one, examining the mechanics of my life, from relearning guitar to juggling to opening this bottle.

For example, I realized that to relearn the guitar when I couldn't play a note required the patience to play scales over and over again; that mustering the will to learn the D-chord took the patience of a saint for months at a time. When I began learning guitar at ten years old, I studied chord charts and repeated these painstaking and boring scales until I could take no more, but I had never *fully* learned them. I gave up and settled for less.

Wondering how many other things I'd blown off in my life, my mind plowed through years of history in a matter of seconds. This was it: I was no longer satisfied with how I used to live and learn. My life was now different and forever changed, and I was now a different person.

I sat down on a ledge and put in the necessary time to get the bottle open the right way. It was still a struggle to envision and then actually accomplish removing the cap, but I did it. I drank a long, cool draft of water. Then I ran back to the stage and hugged Barb exuberantly.

"Babe," I blurted, "I just had a revelation. I used to accept less, but now have much higher expectations. The stroke forced me to slow down, and it helped me apply one hundred percent of myself to every task. Things that confounded me must now be met head-on. I refuse to accept my inabilities without giving them my all. My world has changed."

I couldn't get it out fast enough.

Since I didn't have a pen and paper, and my memory was still wanting, I told Barb everything and made her promise to write down her version of my epiphany as soon as we got home. She kissed me, looked in my eyes, and promised that she would do the best she could with her fifty-six-year-old memory. As it turns out, the revelation was so deep and so powerful that I remembered every detail and emotion on my own, and did not need her help to recall it.

It's been many months since that night. I've had time to assess my revelation, and I've seen the changes every day. My NIA and dancing has changed. The transitions between steps and movements have become smoother and less jerky, more rhythmic and natural. My guitar playing, which seemed doomed and impossible to relearn, has become more creative, more melodic, and more enjoyable—though it's still impossible to play at my pre-stroke level. I even penned a song about my stroke. My tennis serve is deadlier than it ever was. I appreciate life more.

My left hand is still numb and continues to be a bit of a dead weight. I still have trouble handling small items. My arm has bouts of tingling and numbness that scare me and elicit flashbacks of my TIAs. I have to talk myself through these feelings and remind myself that the last CT angiogram showed clean arteries and an accepted stent. It may take years before I have full use of my left hand. In the event that it does not return to normal, I will learn to function as is and consider myself lucky for what I *do* have.

I've found that it's best to put off life-changing decisions for six months to a year following a stroke, as I know that mine influenced my heart and mind. I fell in love with the quaint beach town of Encinitas during our stay there, for example, and would have moved there in a blink if we could have sold our Boulder house quickly enough. When I went back to Encinitas just three months later, feeling better and stronger and more confident, I could enjoy it for what it was: a beautiful little town with lots of promise and a great place to visit. But I also knew that Boulder was still the right place for us.

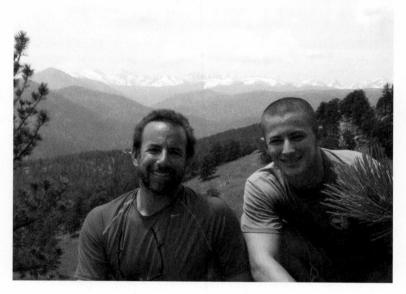

The author with his son Ben

My Sons' Letters to Me

Ben, age 22 (He was with me on the slope the day of the ski accident.):

> I was shocked initially, like what the hell! Then I felt a bit helpless, not because I thought you were doomed, but rather because I couldn't be there [for the surgery]. I was sad, but that wasn't the predominant emotion. I guess it was just a shock. Then the feeling of, "How could this happen to *you*?" (Not just my Dad, but *you*.)
>
> After you'd already had the surgery, I felt sort of fortunate in a bizarre way that I wasn't there, because I didn't want to have to see you like that. Of course I wanted to

see you, but I didn't want to see you *that* way. You and Ma have always been so healthy and haven't suffered the problems of others your age. I had never seen either of you completely vulnerable or really hurt, so it would have greatly affected me to see you like that.

I worried about the risk of the surgery, even though I thought it would be fine. When you were in the surgery and Ma said you should be out in a half hour, I called on the half hour until you were out, but you were in for two hours. I was at a friend's place, but I couldn't stop thinking about it.

I thought of you never having been one to complain or have a lack of willpower or discipline when it counts.

Bryan, age 25:

I didn't cry. I felt overwhelmed and amazed. I remember growing up, always feeling like you were bulletproof. You would step on a bee and not flinch. Twist an ankle and just grit your teeth. Go in for surgery on the cyst behind your knee, and just take it as any other aspect of life. That may have been the truth, or it may have been a facade as a means of internalizing your fears in front of us. But this time was different. There was no covering your fears or hesitation.

I remember the numerous sprained ankles I suffered through years of basketball. Mom would be so empathetic, and you would just say, "Walk it off." This made it harder for me to accept that what you were undergoing was as serious as it was.

I think the part that scared me the most was the mental aspect. I didn't like, nor did I want to accept, that you were hindered mentally. I was afraid that it could potentially become a permanent condition. When I spoke to you for the first time, from your hospital bed, I felt relieved that your memory was mostly intact. You were far from 100% coherent, and it was obvious that you weren't able to define your emotions by the same means you could previously. It was strange for me to witness you struggle to find the words that came to you so easily just two days earlier. But I was still reassured by the words you did say, and I was cautiously optimistic about what the future held. Regardless, it did consume my thoughts for a few days, especially during the five days before you were released from the hospital. I remember drinking six beers by myself—the night Mom called me—before I was able to talk to you.

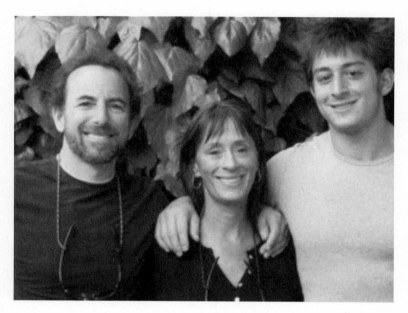

The author with his wife, Barb, and their son Bryan

Support Groups

I attended my first support meeting for stroke survivors in November of 2008. A social worker and a therapist had organized the meeting. I highly recommend attending a meeting or two along with your partner or caregiver, even if you think that you're not a "group" kind of person, or you feel like you're "past all that."

Most of the survivors seemed pleased to be there. People enjoyed cookies and drinks as everyone mingled. A local neurologist spoke for thirty minutes about different therapies and supplements, followed by a brief question-and-answer period. After the doctor left there were introductions and updates by all the attendees. I found it very loose and easy, and it provided a great opportunity to schmooze and learn. In the months and years since then, I've been very active in this and other survivors' groups.

Postscript: May 2011

I was just invited to speak at my stroke support group meeting this October!

Marijuana

With regard to smoking pot during my rehabilitation, I do want to share a few additional thoughts. Smoking at that critical time in my life helped me see outside myself and to reach new heights that I could not attain given my own inertia. Most importantly, it helped me "see the light" during an otherwise dark and depressing period of my recovery. I used it to break out and find new ways of seeing things that I couldn't achieve on my own. I reached thresholds that might have taken weeks, months, or even years to attain—or may not have been attainable at all without this catalyst and inspiration.

After reaching these pinnacles and achieving increased awareness, as well as a greater degree of mobility, I also reached a place of peace within myself and have continued to draw on these strengths and achievements without smoking pot.

A Realization About Others: The Peace That Passeth Understanding

I've noticed a phenomenon common to most of the stroke survivors I interviewed, whom you will meet in the next section. Of the fourteen men and women, from twenty-two to sixty-seven years of age, the majority stated—quite emphatically—that they do not regret the experience and would *not* reverse the effects of stroke, regardless of their cognitive deficits. I do believe, however, that each of these people would do almost anything to get their physical abilities back.

You may think that in an effort to make the best of a bad situation, these people are deceiving themselves. But I beg to differ. Just as I have experienced a calm that has washed over me, many of these survivors have been infused with comfort and peace, too. Perhaps that's why they are satisfied with their current condition. Maybe that's why they believe that the experiences, the lessons learned, and the people they've met have made the stroke worthwhile.

Most of the people I interviewed believe that this new inner state of mind is a better place to be, regardless of how they got there. People who have not experienced stroke or some similar brain trauma cannot really relate to this phenomenon, and may consider this acceptance to be a cop-out—just a way of escaping reality. Granted, it may seem a convenient way to leave the rat race, but stroke survivors have their own hell to deal with.

The next questions may be: Are these survivors even cognizant of where they were in the first place versus where they are now? Are they aware of what has transpired? Maybe they lack the ability to recognize that things *are* different, and they just like where they are now.

Most of the interviewees recall who they used to be, and how they used to be, and say they are much happier where they are now and would not trade it back. Frivolous things that once seemed important are now less pressing. Personally, I refuse to be rushed or intimidated, and I refuse to submit to the stress that occasionally dictated my life. When someone pressures me beyond reason, I tell him or her, "I cannot be pressured and I will not stress over it." Am I using the stroke as an excuse to escape the pressures of reality? Or have I seen the light and gravitated toward it? Is it possible that what we know now is what we should have known from the start?

In my case, I have regained most of my physical abilities and I am still working to regain the cognitive loss, but I am happy with my newfound disposition and I would not give back my stroke, even if I could.

Perhaps if you are a newly recovering stroke survivor, you will find this hard to believe. But I am proud and happy to tell you that it's only a matter of time and practice before you discover a better version of yourself, for yourself.

I wish you strength, hope, and joy as you embark on your healing.

PART TWO

INTERVIEWS WITH STROKE SURVIVORS

INTERVIEWS WITH
STROKE SURVIVORS

Iwas not able to begin these interviews until nine months after my stroke, and it took another three months to edit them. But after conducting these interviews and getting to know so many inspiring stroke survivors, I came to a number of conclusions.

Almost all of the interviewees have undergone permanent change as a result of their stroke. Some did eventually go back to work, in the same capacity, but most either left their life's vocation after a short period or did not return to it at all. Some changed their jobs because they could not perform as they did in their pre-stroke days. In many cases, these people were so affected by the stroke that they focused their energy on helping survivors and other disabled people through support groups and volunteer work.

When I finally became well enough to reach out to other stroke survivors, I found their stories fascinating. I found a common thread among the survivors I interviewed: They all expressed an interest and a pleasure in hearing my story *and* sharing theirs. I never thought I would be so intrigued by accounts of other peoples' stroke experiences, but, once they started telling their stories, I realized how strong our bond really was. I also found that not all, but many, had a great sense of humor in the telling of their stroke experience.

Each person openly shared highly personal tales of their struggles and cared little about anonymity. Though most survivors still live with the effects of their stroke, it took effort for them to summon up the memories of their early experiences, as well as the courage needed to recount them, and I thank them wholeheartedly for that effort. I caught up with some of them again a year after our original interviews; their stories have been updated. In addition, spouses and partners of survivors have to endure incredible upheaval and change when nursing and supporting their loved ones. They are often the unsung heroes and silent sufferers in these life-changing experiences. So, I asked the survivors for permission to interview their partners and spouses, and most agreed to chat, so I have included a special section on spouses and partners, as well.

GARY

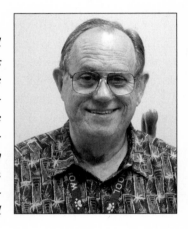

Gary is a thoughtful and focused sixty-three-year-old. He had his stroke at fifty-six, and has made an impressive recovery after spending a full month in a coma. Like some of our other survivors, he suffered a hemorrhagic stroke, which in his opinion could have been avoided if he'd been more diligent about treating his high blood pressure.

I was working on the computer at home around 10 AM when the cursor on the screen stopped working. I messed with it for about fifteen minutes, and then realized that it was not the mouse or the cursor; my arm wouldn't work right. I called my brother, who suggested that I go next door and see my neighbor, who's a doctor. I was on the second floor and had a very hard time getting down the stairs. I don't drink, but felt like I was drunk and disoriented. I made it down without falling. But before I could get to my neighbor's door, the doctor came running out (my brother had called him), and then the paramedics pulled up. I can't even say that I knew what a stroke was.

At some point I lost consciousness and fell into a coma. Weeks later, I woke to the Rose Parade on TV, which I recognized by some of the events and landmarks. I watched it for a few minutes, perhaps ten or more. I thought they were speaking another language, maybe Spanish. Later I found out that it was English, I just couldn't comprehend what they were saying. Then I went back into the coma and woke again, permanently, a week or two later. My family was gathered around because they had just disconnected the ventilator and were waiting for me to die. Apparently, disconnecting the ventilator shocked me out of the coma and jump-started my system. It could have gone either way, I guess.

I thought it was the day after I arrived at the ER. And I thought I was in San Antonio, Texas, but I was in Long Beach, California. I was like that for about a week. You could draw a line down the center of my body, from my head to my groin: I couldn't feel anything on the right side. I couldn't even tell it was there. The left side of my body was completely fine and everything worked. But I *was* right-handed, so I was completely incapable of doing the simplest things. I couldn't walk, talk, write, or feed myself.

I was somewhat aware of my condition, but I didn't care. I just lay there in a fog. For the whole first week, I was oblivious and disinterested. I thought I could speak and be understood. I could make noise, but everything I said was unintelligible. It took me two months to be able to speak basic words. However, about two weeks after I came out of the coma, my relatives brought my sixteen-year-old nephew to visit, and that made all the difference. Jeff is deaf, and he could actually understand much of what I was saying, so he became my translator.

My doctor would come to my room each morning and ask me my name and the date. I knew my name and wondered why he kept asking me that. But not knowing the date pissed me off, so I asked my relatives to bring me a large calendar.

They tacked it to the wall, and each day they would cross off the date so I could keep up. When the doctor came and asked me the date, I would sneak a look at the calendar before answering. I did this for a few days, and then he congratulated me, without knowing that I'd cheated. That was the first time after the stroke that I cared about anything.

My cognitive improvement was gradual. When they worked with me on my language, the therapist said, "Dick bought two pair of shoes and Jane bought two pair of shoes. How many shoes did Dick and Jane buy?" I had no idea. I realized quickly that I couldn't add or subtract or read, and I was literally sobbing. I realized then that I had some big problems.

One day, about two months or so into my stay, I was working in the therapy room and all of sudden I found myself in the corner crying. I felt that I wasn't accomplishing anything, which made me feel like a complete failure. They discovered that I had not been given my Ritalin that day. They gave it to me, and I felt normal an hour later. They had prescribed Ritalin as an experiment, and it made a huge difference. After that, everything was better.

My relatives were adamant that I start rehab as soon as possible, but the doctors did not expect much improvement. They figured that they'd put me in rehab for a week and then send me to a rest home.

The physical therapist would lay me on a table and ask me to kick her hand with my right foot, and I could only move it about an inch. We did this every day. But one day my leg moved about twelve inches, and I kicked her square in the face! She got up without a word and ran out of the room. I sat there feeling bad, afraid that I had hurt her and was now in trouble.

She came back with a group of therapists and asked me to kick again, which I did, gladly. They were all very excited, and it was at this point that they changed their tune and started committing themselves to my rehab. It was a big moment for me. I figured that between the Ritalin and my newfound physicality, I was on the way to recovery and would be home in a week. Of course, I was delusional; delusional, but happier.

In the long run, I'd work for five days on something with little improvement, and then on the sixth day I could do it. That was a distinct pattern: no change, no change, and then: *Ooh!* A very noticeable change. And that was very encouraging.

I could stand up and walk a little by the time I left rehab, but they would not let me use a walker because of the limited strength on my left side, so I rolled out of rehab in a wheelchair. My right side, as a whole, was much the same. I could stand and put weight on my right leg, but do very little with it. Eight years later, it's still like that. If I want the right side to do something, I have to tell it in detail to do it; it does not come automatically to me. If I want to move my right arm to the right side of the wheelchair, I have to tell it where to position and how far back to go. If I use my right side for something and get distracted in the process, the right side will literally fall or become lame. It takes constant vigilance.

I had to move from my second-story apartment to a ground floor place, so I took a converted garage/apartment just two blocks from the hospital. Before the hospital released me, they had to inspect the apartment to make sure it had proper wheelchair access. They also required me to have a caregiver, at least in the morning, to help me dress and prepare food. I hired a caregiver, who was a part-time nurse at the hospital, but she never showed up. That first morning was a fiasco; I spent over three hours just getting dressed and making breakfast. But I never told the hospital. From that point on I learned to support myself; very slowly, but surely! And it did get better.

I also did outpatient therapy for about three years following my stroke. I learned how to tie my shoe with one hand and to shave with my "wrong" hand, which was a bloody mess until I could get a handle on it. It's amazing what a strong will and stubbornness will help you achieve!

In terms of therapy, I had regular massages and electric stimulation. I did not have acupuncture, but some of my stroke-survivor friends have used it and felt it was helpful. I have a friend who did water therapy and he said it was very helpful.

Before the stroke, I was a fat, lethargic person. I weighed 280 pounds, did very little exercise, ate three or four steaks a week, and ate a lot of restaurant food. It was the perfect diet to have a stroke or a heart attack! To save money on blood pressure medication, I'd skip days or cut down the dosage; it caused massive fluctuations, which can be more dangerous than having constant high blood pressure. This eventually led to my stroke.

Do I blame myself? Not really. It is what it is, and I am who I am. Life's too short to worry over such things.

It sounds dumb for a stroke survivor in a wheelchair to say this, but I feel better than I did before the stroke. I am thinner, and I am mentally happier and more balanced than I ever was. I had lost almost eighty pounds by the time I left rehab, which certainly helped me acclimate to life outside. I purposely don't use a motorized wheelchair so I can move my blood and get *some* exercise. My wheelchair is made of titanium, which is very lightweight and easy to load and unload from my van, and that process provides a little exercise as well.

Oddly enough, I do not look at myself any differently than I do anyone else. Everyone has problems in their life, something that hangs them up. So I'm in a wheelchair—so what? I have my van. I've been able to maintain a sense of humor; I always make jokes about myself. True, I can't go back to work because of my fatigue level. I can "run" until noon, but then need my hour-long nap. But between my support group, my work at the library, my volunteer work at the VA and St. Mary's Hospital, board meetings, and church on Sunday, I live a very active life.

. . . Honestly, neither the physical nor the cognitive challenges have been particularly hard. I have never said, "Why me? Why did this happen?" I was depressed in the beginning, and the Ritalin helped, but I just don't have many complaints. From the moment I came out of the coma I've been glad to be alive. The only thing that I can't do now is ride my motorcycle.

The VA paid for all my medical expenses and rehabilitation. They also cover my medicine and prescriptions based on my ability to pay. In my case, since I live on disability, I am fully covered. The VA was my first support group, and they have been most helpful. I still go to that weekly. After I got my driver's license back, I was asked to be on the Board of the Southern California Stroke Association. I liked those meetings very much and continue to go, and actually help run the place.

When I first got out of in-patient rehab, I just stayed at home and went to physical therapy. I was in a wheelchair, feeling self-conscious and internalized. The VA support group finally convinced me to go out to a large shopping mall, and I was quite surprised that no one paid me any mind. That trip to the mall did wonders for me. It was a great relief to be part of the real world again.

I am now left-handed because my right hand doesn't work. I have no choice. I only use my right hand to hold things down. I type most correspondence on the computer—albeit slowly—because my handwriting is atrocious. The one thing I was worried about was my signature for the bank, but they took my check anyway! Some people are quite amazed that I can do things like tie my shoe with one hand. I give myself an extra point for originality.

Would I reverse the whole stroke experience if I had the chance? No, not in a million years. What I have accomplished cannot be replaced. My life is much nicer now. I don't worry as much, and I appreciate and enjoy what I have. My apartment is small and my van is close to twenty years old, but I'm okay with that. Before the stroke, I put too much effort and thought into cars and houses. I don't have those issues now and I don't miss them. It's a nice peaceful life. I would like the ability to walk freely and enjoy the luxuries that come with being "normal," but given the things I've learned, I would definitely go with life *after* the stroke.

JAMIE

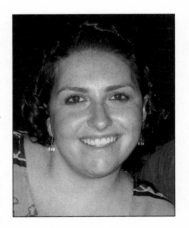

Jamie was twenty-two when she had her stroke. She had just graduated from college and was in a celebratory mood, looking forward to finding a job and moving on. She is now twenty-three.

I had a killer headache for about two days, so I finally went to the hospital. They couldn't find anything conclusive and sent me home. I returned twice more over the course of several days. The third time they did a CT scan, but still found nothing, so they gave me a boatload of pills. Back at home, I couldn't stand up, and collapsed onto the couch.

I called my father, who flew in immediately. When he showed up at my apartment, I was naked. I was twenty-two, and I did *not* want to be naked in front of my father. I told him that I couldn't find my clothes, yet there was clothing everywhere. From there I got progressively worse.

When they tried to do an MRI in the emergency room, I was screaming and combative. I even said to my dad, "Who are you? Get the fuck away from me!" My father called a few of my friends to help calm me down, but I cussed at them as well. I told them to stop screaming when they were actually whispering. The ER doctor called the neurologist, who apparently suggested that they knock me out so they could do the MRI.

The MRI showed that the central vein in my brain was totally clotted. I had suffered something called cerebral venous sinus thrombosis, or CVST, a rare form of stroke that results from a clot in the dural venous sinuses, causing blood to drain from the brain.

I have no memory until I woke up from a coma twelve days later. Even with heparin thinning my blood, my inner-cranial pressure was so high while I was comatose that they were worried my brain was going to herniate into the brain stem, which could have left me totally brain-dead. They thought a craniotomy (a surgical procedure to remove part of the skull to access the brain) would take care of it, but they ended up having to do a second one a few days later.

I didn't understand what had happened. I had crazy, bizarre dreams while I was in the coma and wasn't sure, even days later, what was reality and what was a dream. All I know was that I craved a burger and fries, that my head was bald, and that I had tubes in my arms and tubes coming out of my head. I just wanted to get out of the hospital and hang out with friends and have a few beers. I had no idea how severe my condition was.

I came out of the coma with very few side effects; no paralysis, no facial distortion, and no visual problems. My right side was a bit weaker than my left, but that improved in a matter of hours. I did have trouble putting thoughts together and pretty bad short-term memory. They bombard you with speech, occupational, cognitive, and physical therapy within hours of stabilizing, but most of that was fine. What I really needed was talk therapy. Psychologically, I was not okay for a long while.

I spent three months in the hospital, most of it in the ICU. When I was well enough, I did some time in a rehab center. I mostly bitched about being in the hospital. I was not a happy camper, and I just wanted out.

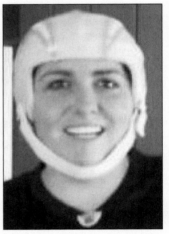

When I left the hospital I could walk and move my limbs, but I was very fatigued and had to be extremely careful not to fall and hurt my head. I didn't have my skull back on, so I wore a hard helmet to protect the soft tissue on my exposed brain. I ordered a special helmet in pink, and my boyfriend bought me San Diego Charger lightning bolts to put on it. I tried to have fun with it, but it wasn't fun at all—but what are you going to do?

My lease actually ran out while I was in the coma, so my parents and friends packed up my apartment, and my parents rented a house nearby. So I actually moved "home" into my parents' house, which is not exactly how I envisioned living after graduation.

I was tired, and even though I was allowed to remove the helmet to lie down, I couldn't get comfortable and didn't sleep well. I pretty much just sat around and felt sorry for myself. My friends would come over, but they were busy interviewing for jobs and going to football games, which is what I should have been doing. Instead I'd had two craniotomies and a shunt placement, and I was just biding my time till returning to the hospital for cranioplasty, a procedure to reset that piece of my skull back over my brain.

It took me about four months to admit that I was *extremely* depressed and to start dealing with it. I was seeing my therapist twice a week, but I spent most of my time crying. As I look back now, I realize that I was grieving. I had lost the carefree person I once was. My friends were all moving forward and I was having a hard time getting dressed in the morning. It was like, "What's the point of getting up or taking a shower?" I had nothing to do and no place to go.

I was fed up with living with my parents, so I sent them home and moved in with my boyfriend. He was working full-time, and I just sat on the couch. About four months after my stroke, I started on antidepressants and joined a gym, and that became my daily routine for another four months. Most of my friends had all but disappeared. They were of the mind that this thing—once I recovered physically—was like a broken bone. "You're healed, so let's go out and party." They don't understand that being in a really noisy place or going clubbing is not really my first choice of activities these days. When I finally healed from the severe depression of the stroke and the recovery, I became depressed about losing my friends.

I did some body massage to help me relax because I was hyper-vigilant all the time. I still have real trouble organizing and remembering things. I've taken to color-coding my daily calendar so I don't miss appointments. I also saw a Hakomi therapist, from Naropa Institute. She focused on the physiological signs that my body was giving me. I'm now working part-time and I'm thinking of attending Naropa to get a degree in counseling.

While there's no clear evidence that my stroke was the result of being on birth control pills for the last six years before my stroke, I do believe that they are the reason it happened. Some of my neurologists and hematologists agreed. Stroke *is* a known possible side effect, and there are many reported cases. I'm off birth control pills and I also take the blood thinner, so I don't really fear having another stroke. I still have a shunt in place in case I do. I'd hope that they wouldn't have to shave my head. I know that sounds shallow, but losing my hair was very traumatic. I am still angry about the stroke and the brain surgeries. I feel more like a victim than a survivor, and I've learned that re-victimization is quite common.

The hospital bill was over a million dollars. I exhausted my insurance, drained my family's savings, and might have to file for bankruptcy—and I don't even know what that means. I'm twenty-three and have never been in touch with income tax and all that. My father handled the paperwork and arranged payment for my bills. I am very concerned about my financial future but, honestly, I can't really deal with it yet.

Since the stroke, I've become tighter with my family. My mother is my hero; she never left my side. I am truly touched by the support they showed during this whole thing, and I appreciate them much more. I am also very thankful for my boyfriend, Shane. He has been a huge support through it all! I have also matured a lot. I believe that this experience has shown me a clearer path to my future, and I'm excited about exploring a career in counseling. I realize how precious time really is, and I now choose to use it wisely. I've had to sit on my deathbed.

Postscript: May 2011

I will most likely be on blood thinners for life, but other than that my health is stellar. The doctors continue to be shocked by my recovery. I feel fortunate to be able-bodied after what I survived. I am completing my Masters degree in transpersonal psychology and starting my internship, which really feels like the beginning of my career. For the first time since I was burdened with my health catastrophe I am now a normal 26-year-old woman, and all the pieces are coming together!

STEPHEN

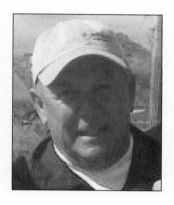

Stephen is sixty-two. He had his stroke just months before this interview, caused by a blockage from plaque in the right carotid artery that resulted in left-side paralysis. He's a spry guy, full of energy and gusto, and he uses his positive energy to cheerlead other stroke survivors on to greater heights.

I was alone at home one morning, just strolling to the kitchen. Suddenly I lost all strength in my body and fell to the floor like a sack of bricks. I got back up five or six times and actually drove to meet my kids for dinner that night. I never said a word to my family about what was going on. I didn't even go to the doctor until the next day; that's how stupid I was.

My brother-in-law took me to the doctor. I could barely walk, so he tried to help support me. The thing is, he doesn't walk very well either, and we fell a few times in the parking lot. We had to solicit the help of another guy in the parking lot to get me back up! I spent an hour with the doctor, who had my brother-in-law drive me to the ER as soon as we were done. My left side was completely paralyzed. My vision and speech were good, and I had no facial droop. I wasn't exactly disoriented, but I could not focus on the task at hand.

I wasn't exactly aware of the signs of stroke before having mine. In terms of my pre-stroke health and fitness, I was probably about a seven-and-a-half out of ten. I was working out a few times a week with a professional trainer. I had quit smoking about six months before as part of my regimen, but I was still overdoing the cheeseburgers and Coke.

One doctor followed the next, and they all told me what a fool I was for waiting so long to come in. They found a small clot in the brain. I spent two weeks in the VA hospital, but they did only about a week of physical therapy. Then I was transferred to a rehabilitation hospital for five weeks, where I did about three hours of PT every day. I also did occupational therapy. My speech was fine, so they focused on my cognitive issues, giving me tests to determine my ability to read and decipher rows of images, like rabbits and such.

They worked on my left arm and shoulder, which had virtually no movement. They did the peg-in-the-hole test, and I couldn't lift my shoulder to put even one peg in the hole. My fingers worked the whole time, however, and I had pretty good tensile strength in my left hand.

I'll never forget the breakthrough I had one Saturday while watching a football game on TV. I was supporting my arm in the up position, and all of a sudden I got the use of my arm back and it stayed up there on its own. I said, "Holy shit, this is excellent!" Two weeks later, my twin brother goaded me into using the walker. I told him that I didn't have the strength and I wasn't ready yet. This was less than two weeks before I got out of the hospital. But I started working hard on the walker, and before I knew it I was walking all over the freaking hospital. It was monumental. I will never forget that day. I eventually graduated to walking with a four-prong cane with a support belt for safety.

My right side never had any issues, which is fortunate since I'm right-handed. The coordination in my left hand is about a four on a scale of ten, and my strength is about the same. My left shoulder is still very weak and spastic, and I do outpatient PT two times a week. The range of motion is not too bad, but it's not very coordinated. My leg is probably a seven. My cognitive capacity and ability to focus is around a five. I have always been impatient, and it's worse now, so I don't expect major improvement in that area. I learned all the rudiments of cooking, showering, and cleaning in the rehab hospital and now do most of that on my own. I still take the walker with me when I leave the house, but I never use it. I work very hard with my typing and have decent finger control, but my shoulder makes even the simplest process challenging. I get lazy and have to force myself to use the left hand and not cheat. I squeeze a putty ball at every opportunity. I get very fatigued and take naps every afternoon, but don't wake up all that refreshed.

My state of mind following the stroke was not bad. The nurses and the rehabilitation staff said that I set the record for the most phone calls and the most visitors. Mentally and emotionally I had a lot of support, and I had a positive attitude from the start. I was always a happy-go-lucky guy, and I remained that way during this whole experience. I didn't struggle with depression the way many stroke survivors do. My psychologist at the rehab was drop-dead beautiful, a *ten,* so I was never depressed in her presence! Now, if I'd been told that I'd never play golf again, then I would have been depressed. I am passionate about my golf, and I've been out twice since I got out of the hospital. It's still very early in my rehabilitation, but I hope to get ninety percent of my physicality back.

I *have* experienced something of a personality change. If I tell a joke or if I hear something funny, I will laugh uncontrollably until I cry. I even cry when I watch sentimental commercials! If you take me to a chick flick I'll be asking for Kleenex, and that was *never* the case before my stroke. I was always a bulletproof hard-ass. I think it's more funny than not. I have these laughing fits in front of friends, and it's a little embarrassing, but I can deal with it.

The one thing I'm scared about is the possibility of having another stroke. I know that I was lucky this time. I'll find out more when I meet with the doctor about putting a stent in my carotid. I was never on Plavix or Coumadin, but I take an aspirin a day and I'm on a cholesterol drug. I'm hoping that my improved diet will take care of the high cholesterol and get me off those meds.

If I had the chance to reverse the whole stroke and rehabilitation experience, I would.

DINA

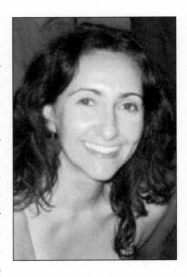

Dina was thirty years old when she had her stroke seven years ago. Her story is different than most because her paralysis and associated symptoms resolved themselves in three hours; she was able to "walk" out of the hospital after a week of emotional and physical turmoil. However, Dina still experienced the horrors of stroke and the subsequent stress of continued treatment. Interestingly, she is a trained physical therapist and has worked with many stroke survivors before and since her stroke.

I was in a morning Pilates class with a friend when I started feeling woozy. I tried to drink some water and couldn't swallow. I had slurred speech and couldn't move my left arm. I could move my left leg, but it wasn't a controlled movement. Cognitively, I was totally aware of everything that was happening. My classmates immediately called 911.

The ride to the hospital was very surreal. The paramedic was calling my case in to the ER, saying, "Possible thirty-year-old stroke . . ." I knew he was talking about me, but it felt foreign and impossible, like an out-of-body experience. Being in the health-care field, and knowing what the potential results could be, I was very scared.

In the ER, I was surrounded by a team of doctors and nurses pulling off my shirt and pants, inserting an IV line, telling me to straighten my arm when I couldn't. The doctor held up my arm and told me to keep it there, but it was dead and just flopping around. My speech was slurred as I tried talking to my hand and arm, commanding them to move.

I was going through it, but didn't feel that I was a part of it. My friend was with me, which helped calm me, but I'd been completely healthy an hour before and would never have imagined myself in this position. Here I was, a patient for the first time in my life! On the gurney ride up to radiology, I thought about my condition and what would happen if the paralysis were permanent. In my head I was still talking to my body, telling it to move. My fear was mounting when, out of nowhere, I felt some movement in the fingers of my left hand. I was elated. My faculties started returning during the ride back from radiology to the ER, which calmed me to no end. I could move my arm, my speech returned, and I just had some numbness and tingling in my left hand. But even after the majority of the symptoms had resolved, I could only think about what might have been.

I worked at a rehab facility in a medical center, so I asked to be transferred there. I was admitted to the Neurology unit. They scheduled me for a TEE (transesophageal echocardiogram) to see if I had a hole in my heart. The results were positive. I had a small hole called a PFO (patent foramen ovale). The test also revealed an ASA (atrial septal aneurysm). This is a thinning of the wall between the two upper chambers of the heart. The little opening allows clots to pass through the heart and travel to the brain. The PFO and ASA are congenital abnormalities, neither of which I previously knew about.

A nurse came into my room wanting to give me Coumadin and start me on a heparin drip. I refused to take it without speaking to the doctor myself. He said that he had told me about starting on the Coumadin after having the TEE, but

I had no memory of that. I was shocked by the presumption on their part—even coming from the health-care field myself. Being on the patient side of things was a real shot of reality, and not a very pleasant one. The doctor did explain that this was a typical protocol for a PFO, and I was then started on Coumadin to minimize the chance of another clot. The day had started with the stroke at 9 AM and it ended with the TEE results at 9 PM, so it was a long day. I couldn't sleep, so I did yoga on the floor of my room in an attempt to relieve my stress and center myself.

The next day I had an MRI, which revealed a clot in the basal ganglia part of my brain. The MRI confirmed that I had had a stroke, but they still didn't know what caused it. I was young and healthy and there was no history of stroke in my family. However, I had started on birth control pills three months before, which increases clotting—though the chance of having a stroke is supposed to be minimal.

I stayed at the medical center for six days because they couldn't regulate my Coumadin to a therapeutic level. While there, I consulted with many physicians regarding whether to repair the hole or remain on Coumadin. A recent study had revealed a higher incidence of cryptogenic stroke (meaning a stroke of unknown origin) in younger people; and people who have PFOs *and* an atrial septal aneurysm are at a higher risk of having a second stroke compared to people with just a PFO.

I decided to stay on Coumadin until more research surfaced. There was a huge study being done that compared the prolonged use of Coumadin versus doing a PFO repair. I waited, having regular checkups to monitor my blood levels. This is a strong drug and I was very young and extremely active, so it was stressful and scary. I bruised very easily and had to watch what I ate. I was on Coumadin for three years and then decided to have my hole repaired.

I took an intellectual approach—blocking out the emotional side while I started gathering information. This was "my" hospital, where I worked, so I knew a number of the staff members. It was a teaching hospital and I was a "thirty-year-old stroke," so a lot of the doctors wanted to work on my case. I tried to appreciate the attention, but I felt like a piece of meat, which really pissed me off.

I wanted to see my MRI report, so a doctor took me into a room to view it. While I was there, another doctor came into the room and said, "Oh, you're the thirty-year-old stroke. You're lucky that the clot wasn't a little to the left." I told the chief resident that I was appalled by this doctor's bedside manner, and he spoke to the resident about this, which helped, but I was bitter. You really have to be your own advocate at every step.

I went to stay with my parents for two weeks after getting out of the hospital. I was a wreck, mentally and emotionally. I laid around in a depressed trance, feeling sorry for myself, asking why this happened to me. I did some yoga and I ran a few miles a few times, but I was afraid of running too long a distance. Not knowing the cause of the stroke put me in a dark place.

I went back to work roughly three weeks after the stroke. But the possibility of having another stroke consumed my thoughts. Every headache, every perceived feeling of tingling or numbness was a sign—all probably aggravated by anxiety.

Eventually I decided to have the hole in my heart repaired. I was thinking about getting married and having kids, and I could not have kids while taking Coumadin. The hole could also have presented issues because of the pressure that birthing puts on the heart. I thought it was time to do it, and I'm glad I did. I didn't end up marrying the guy, but when it's time to have kids I will be ready.

At work, I was treating a forty-year-old man who'd had a stroke around the same time I did, and coincidentally also had a PFO. I ended up having my procedure done by the same interventional cardiologist that did his repair. You go in for the appointment and the doctor shows you these devices sitting on a table, and you're imagining them inside your heart; it's a very strange and disconcerting experience. I wanted to know everything, so there I was watching a video on the procedure before I had the procedure. Sometimes too much information is not a good thing. There's still that emotional component, and I was reeling from it.

But it was a simple procedure, done through a catheter, and I now have a titanium and nickel device for PFO closures, sitting between the two upper chambers of my heart. I was awake and watched the whole thing on a monitor. In my mind there were no more questions; the decision had been made. I went in with a sense of tranquility and came home the following day. Thank God it all went well.

My life is starting to get back to normal. It's a new normal, but everything is back in place and running smoothly. I've run four marathons and have learned to deal with it all. I wanted to start a group for young survivors, but I had no idea how to start the group or how to structure it once it got going. One of the senior social workers offered to run the group with me, so we've been co-leading this young persons' group for over two years. It is a great outlet for everyone, and the exchange of information and the sharing of experiences are invaluable. No matter how much a spouse or partner or relative says they understand a person's condition, no one can understand as much as a fellow stroke survivor. Everyone supports each other.

I am also very involved with the National Stroke Association and have run the New York City Marathon to raise money. And I'm an active member of the Young Professionals Group of the American Heart and American Stroke Association and give talks and do interviews to raise awareness.

Would I rather have not had a stroke? Yes. But would I give up the relationships I've established or the opportunities to help others that have come as a result of it? No. I believe that everything in life happens for a reason. Perhaps this is a way of rationalizing unpleasant events that occur in my life, but whatever the motivation, I believe that having a stroke was in my cards.

MARK

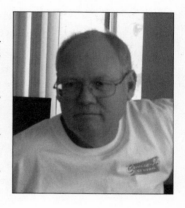

Mark was forty when he had his stroke; he is now fifty-three. He had a "catastrophic" stroke—left brain, right side. Like some of the other survivors I've interviewed, he's endured his condition for many years without much improvement. He speaks slowly and deliberately. His wife, Diane, has been steadfast in her support.

I had a hole in my heart, a PFO, which was the probable cause of my stroke. PFOs account for roughly 2 percent of all strokes. I had the hole repaired eight years later.

I had my stroke when I was alone for just a minute. Diane was Christmas shopping and had no reason to return, but came home at the same moment that I emerged from the bathroom with my stroke in full bloom; apparently the "pushing" involved in using the toilet can put pressure on the hole in the heart. She has no memory of why she was home. She called an ambulance when she saw me walking in circles and slurring my speech.

I was in good shape before the stroke, but I was drinking a lot of beer and was fifteen pounds overweight. I didn't smoke. . . . I had some warning signs, but when you've been healthy your whole life you don't pay much attention to little aches and pains. I can't remember much, other than an eye twitch, some slight blurriness, and a bit of "dry eye." I did have tingling in my right arm a few times three weeks before the stroke. I just thought I had slept on my arm strangely.

I don't remember much about my first few hours in the hospital because my brain had started to swell, so it took a few days for details to start coming back. I do remember refusing care because I couldn't compute the information the doctors and nurses were sharing. Diane took over, saying that I needed to do what the doctors suggested. We talked briefly about TPA (a "clot buster"), but they did not have any at this emergency room. I was very hungry and asked for a glass of milk. I know they did a battery of tests, but I couldn't name them. I spent most of the day in the ER and was then moved to a regular room.

I tried to talk, but my speech was gone—at least what they could decipher. A few days later I could say yes and no, but I'd say yes when I meant to say no. I still have that problem, so I try to think first before speaking. My face drooped, and it took three or four years of work for that to go away. I spent five days in the hospital, where I had a little therapy, but my stroke occurred a few days before Christmas, and it was hard to get anyone's attention.

From there, I went to a rehabilitation center for two weeks. After I got home, Diane took me to outpatient rehab two to three times a week. Friends and relatives thought that I was released too soon, but you know how insurance works.

By the time I went home I could walk a bit, but my right arm was still dead. However, I had been working my arm very hard in my room, after PT, even though I was instructed to rest. I had my own method of rehabilitation: I built myself a "Rehab Arm" to stimulate my

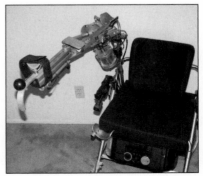

arm, which helped quite a bit. I believe that the arm, elbow, and hand movements are initiated from the armpit. The Rehab Arm, which now has a patent pending, senses which way the arm will go from the cusp of the underarm and fools the brain to feel like it's moving. It makes you feel like you have your arm back, and it brought one man to tears. In fact, the arm has brought two men's arms "back from the dead" after two years, to 50 percent capacity in just three months.

I didn't speak well. I was at maybe 10 percent capacity. I'd go to the refrigerator when I was hungry, point, and say "Yes" or "No." Then Diane would ask me to verify if I really meant whichever word I'd said. I could say a few other simple words. I spent a lot of time watching TV, but I also worked hard on my body. I walked around the house, without my walker, holding onto walls and chairs for stability, trying to balance myself.

I duct-taped my bad arm to my side to keep it out of harm's way and chopped wood with the other arm. I was told that this was a stupid thing to do and that I should quit immediately, but I continued to do it at a slower pace. If I got a cold or some such malady, it could take weeks or months to get better, so I tried to eat well and stay healthy.

Emotionally, I was pretty stable and positive, and didn't get depressed as they said I would. My cognitive ability was definitely hampered. I felt like I was in a dream, and I had to double-check every move I made. I was probably 60 percent gone at that point. I remember that I worked hard not to mess up.

After the stroke I continued enjoying my three beers each night, looking forward to them as an escape from the constant pain on my right side—until about three weeks ago, when I quit drinking to enroll at a pain clinic to see if I can manage the pain without beer. I still take sleeping pills to help me get some quality rest.

I did acupuncture a few times a week, and I'd say that I saw improvement. I also did biofeedback, and that helped.

My progress was all pretty much at the same rate, but there were times when I'd hear a "pop" in my head and something would change for the better. My doctors couldn't explain it. My father-in-law had a stroke a few years after mine, and he said that he heard the pop, too. After the pop I would have an hour of unusual clarity, followed by maybe 20 percent improvement with my speech and physical deficits.

I still get fatigued, and I can never really tell when it's coming. At times I can do some activities quite fully for an hour or so, but then crash and have to take a nap. The change in weather and season can affect my energy. I have burning pain on my right side and constant itching and dull aching every day. This pain wears me out, so I take regular naps for that, as well. The biofeedback I learned puts me in a trancelike state, which also helps the pain, but it does little for my energy level.

I went back to work after six months. I had my own business, with some very good workers who stuck with me, but it got to a point where I was just too diminished and too fatigued. I started driving after a year without incident, but a few times I had to pull over and rethink the situation. I wasn't sure if the light was red or green and just what was required. To this day, I don't drive a whole lot and I never drive at night unless I must.

My blood pressure pre-stroke was 120/80, as a rule, but nowadays it's high. I've started taking medicine for it. I take about twenty pills a day, half of which are vitamins. I am hoping that it will go down now that I have stopped drinking every day. I'd love to get off the meds. My blood pressure was 200/110 on the day I had my stroke.

I don't think much about having another stroke. My cholesterol and blood pressure are under control, and I never did smoke. Besides, every day is like a bonus. . . . After five years, then eight years, I saw some improvement in my coordination and dexterity. Now it's been twelve years, so I don't expect too much more to change. But I'm really satisfied just to be alive.

I would say the emotional challenges have been the hardest to live with. I've accepted my physical condition for the most part. The hardest part is when you start losing friends. You have to keep your words and sentences simple or people start to believe that *you're* simple, too. I have two real friends who have stayed with me throughout. They know that I'm still the same person, regardless of my speech and slower mind.

The whole experience changed the way I saw disabled people. After the stroke, I started noticing everybody who was walking a little bit weird and I'd ask them about their disability. I have an increased awareness and greater compassion for them and their condition. I kept a journal and wrote about them. After stroke, every move you make reminds you of your condition and how far you've come.

I am always looking for ways to improve. Along the way, I've shared my rehabilitation, tips, and breakthroughs with others. It's a two-way street. Most people put a lot of this behind them after the first two years, but I'm still interested to hear people's stories.

MARVEL

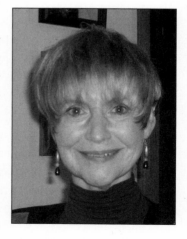

Marvel had her stroke twenty-eight years ago, when she was thirty-four years old. She is now sixty-two, but she still remembers everything; she's lived it over and over again, working with stroke survivors over the past thirty years. Her story reflects the fundamental and somewhat primitive approach toward stroke in 1981 compared to that of today. She is a remarkable woman who's done much work to change the way health-care professionals look at stroke survivors.

I was driving alone when I had a relatively minor car accident; I was, however, knocked unconscious. As a result, the doctors performed a brain scan, which uncovered an arterio-venous malformation (AVM), which is a birth defect that causes a weakening in the blood vessels, resulting in the ballooning of the blood vessel—similar to an aneurysm, but bigger and more complicated. They sent me home after the scan because they felt that the procedure to correct the defect could be deadly, so they did not want to operate. (I didn't learn all this until much later.) They told me to watch for symptoms such as tingling, numbness, or seizures, adding that if I did experience any of these things, I should contact a neurosurgeon right away.

Two years after the accident, I was boating with friends when my left side went so numb that I could have bitten my hand and not felt it. The numbness went away as fast as it came. Had I not known what to look for, I probably would not have gone to the doctor. There are often no symptoms from an AVM, though some people experience the worst headache of their life, and about 60 percent of those die on their way to the hospital. They were still afraid to do the surgery, given the delicacy of the procedure, but I had no choice.

I was in decent health at the time. I took walks, but didn't exercise. I had smoked for years—and continued to smoke even after the stroke. I may have been told to stop smoking, but it was a control issue for me, and the warning didn't register at the time. Then a few years back, I started doing a weekly family health information group with a doctor friend who was very against smoking. After hearing his lectures week after week, I eventually quit. I didn't want to die, especially after I lived through my massive stroke!

I had the AVM surgery about a month after the initial numbness. It lasted eleven hours. They not only had to remove the "ballooned" blood vessel (or "pouch"), but also all the feeder veins. I have about ninety metal clips in my head from the feeder veins they clipped off. The doctor who saved my life is now retired, but he told me that he still has nightmares about the operation. During the procedure they lost control of my vitals because of excessive bleeding, and I suffered a major stroke.

I woke up in the ICU. I remember my sister crying. My face, vision, and voice were fine, but my left side was completely paralyzed. My right side was basically normal; which is fortunate, since I am right-handed. I figured that my deficits would be short-lived. It's not something that you can just accept; like many people, I lived in denial for many years. Cognitively, I thought I was okay. I could converse with friends and family. I didn't really understand the extent of my memory loss until I went back to work.

They started physical therapy every day after I had been moved to the acute care section of the hospital. I couldn't walk and could barely move the left side of my body, but we did some stretching and range-of-motion exercises.

It was like half my body had died and I was in mourning for that half, mourning for what I used to be able to do. I went through all the stages of grief. Everyone goes through that; it's normal. But I had no psychological help because no one told me that I needed it or should seek it. Of course I experienced the denial, the pain, and the "Why me?"s. It's part of the healing process, and it takes a while.

I spent two months with in-patient care and rehabilitation. They worked with my arms and legs. My hand was curled and stiff, but I started getting spastic movement in my arm— which was a good thing. I eventually began walking with a brace and a cane, which shocked them. I remember walking into the outpatient hospital and watching the PT staff jump and shout and applaud. They showed me paperwork stating that I would probably never walk again, but they waited to show me this until *after* I could kind of walk.

Keep in mind that they had removed part of my skull in order to do the surgery, so I was still in a very delicate state. And I was not wearing a helmet as patients do today. I carried on my life in public with a brain just protected by skin—though I did wear scarves and hats. It wasn't until a month later that I went back into the hospital to have an acrylic skull put on. The technology that allows the removal and replacement of the natural bone skull was not available to me at the community hospital.

My first few days at home, I was emotionally distressed. Physically, I had gained weight because I was lying around. But being home was like being let out of jail. Just being able to see the sunshine and go places and see my friends made all the difference; it was the most "normal" I'd felt since the stroke. My high-school-age daughter and my boyfriend were living with me, but she went to school each morning and he went off to work, so I was essentially alone. He did help with meals and other assorted stuff.

I cried every day for a year. I was frustrated and worn out. I was still in PT every day and I lived on the second floor of a non-accessible apartment. I couldn't walk without a brace or a cane and actually had to ascend each stair on my butt, one stair at a time. Plus I'm vain, and I used to be very pretty. I used to wear three-inch spikes to work, and suddenly I couldn't wear any of my favorite shoes. I went eight years without psychological help, and I needed it badly; it just wasn't being offered . . . I was very good at hiding my pain.

However, I did do my PT religiously. I wanted to get better. We also did a lot of OT, and they worked on my cognitive skills. This was a huge rehab hospital, so they had rooms for everything. I could shop in their grocery store, learn how to drive—it was full service . . . I stopped regular PT when I went back to work and felt strong enough to go it alone. I do go back for tune-ups. If you're going to do PT on your own, it's important to make sure that you're doing it correctly. I'll go back to PT every other year to become strong again. I'll do it twice a week for two or three months, or as long as insurance covers it.

I went back to work after a year. I wrote specs for claims-processing systems for Medicare at a major insurance company. They were very understanding and helpful. They gave me the same case file that I was working on before the stroke, but I did not recognize or understand the work, and I had no memory of the acronyms and abbreviations—and in the insurance business there are many. This was the first time I really took stock of how much I had lost from the stroke. I went to the supervisor, closed the office door, and said, "You need to put me back in a training class. I cannot perform at this grade level." I was very lucky; my boss understood, and he put me back in training.

At the time, I attributed my poor performance to being gone for a year, not to my stroke. I was in complete denial; but no doctors told me any different. It was 1982, and the medical profession was still in the Dark Ages with regard to stroke and associated brain injury. There were no neuropsychologists and no neuropsych evaluations offered back then.

I was working downtown, so I would take the train. I kept falling on the train platform and breaking bones. My orthopedic doctor told me that I was going to break my back if I kept up that way. The ice in the winter would have done me in. As a result, I stopped working in 1989 and went on full-time disability.

A short time later, in 1990, after ten years of injury, a neuropsychologist friend referred me to a brilliant doctor. He's triple board-certified in neurology, psychiatry, and is also a physiatrist (physical medicine and rehabilitation). He spent two-and-a-half hours with me on my first visit. I was so impressed with him and the questions he asked. I still see him today.

Overall, I'd say my physical condition today is pretty good, but I have something called left side neglect, which means that I forget it's there. I can move it, but only use it when I have to or when I need two hands. It's not something I remember to use, which is hard for people to understand, but the neglect is part of the injury.

Brain injury is always slow to improve. The physical body does respond and will get better quicker if you work on it diligently. I just don't. I'm tired of working on it, and I openly admit that I could be better if I worked on it, but I've accepted my condition as is. Mentally I am happy, and I'm getting along well. I've been through periods of counseling through the years, and I think it's a good thing to have a professional listen and help occasionally, because they see things that friends and family can't . . . I'm going to say the physical struggle is the worst because it still dogs me, and it will until I die.

For many years, and in many states, people with brain injuries have fallen through the cracks. Many of these people do not qualify for state services because they don't fit the criteria. They may be able to do their ADL ("aid to daily living"), but if their cognitive ability is lacking, then they're screwed. Unless they have a Medicaid brain injury waiver in their state— which we now have here in Illinois because of the work we've been doing—they can't get services, and the state cannot assist them if they qualify for Medicare.

Let's say that you're young and you have a stroke, and you can only qualify for Medicaid. It's hard to get Medicaid if you're walking and talking, but can't think or remember from one minute to the next. If you don't have a brain injury waiver, for any type of brain injury, then you cannot get services. Based on my support group experience, I have found that frontal-lobe injuries can affect your personality, your judgment, and your ability to perceive things accurately, so many of these people with brain injuries face a long uphill battle.

Many people have asked me whether I would take back the stroke if I could. I would not! I have had so many meaningful relationships, so many meaningful projects, and so many meaningful experiences as a result of what's happened to me. I would *never* undo any of this. There are days when I wish it would go away, but I would never wish that it didn't happen because I would not have the life I have and would not have met the people I have if not for this injury.

JOHN

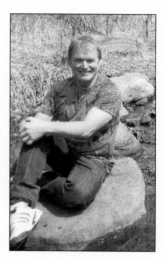

John was forty-four when he had his stroke. He is now fifty-seven. He was visiting from Australia when we met. John was an elite athlete and physical education teacher when he had his stroke. His was yet another incidence of stroke resulting from an accident during physical activity. He is the father of four girls, ages twenty to twenty-eight.

I was in a bike race in October of '95 with over two hundred riders. I was doing about 35 mph when a rider in front of me hit a stick and wiped out. I could not avoid his bike and ran over his wheel. My bike turned in mid-air, and I hit the pavement headfirst. I was wearing a helmet, which may have saved my life, but I took a direct hit to my left side, dislocating my shoulder, whacking the left side of my head, face, and hip, and sustaining three cracks in my helmet. I went to the hospital, where they did an X-ray of the shoulder, but did not do a scan or MRI of anything above my neck. Other than the issues I described above, it was just another fall. I got back on the bike a few weeks later and continued working out and teaching as usual.

On a Saturday night about three months after the bike accident, my wife, Gail, tried to wake me from a deep sleep, but I didn't move. My eyes were open, so she thought I was awake. She slapped my face and I still didn't respond. She called a neighbor to help. He poked me in the ribs and jostled me, but still no movement. I heard them talking and could hear the call they made for an ambulance, but I could not move or speak. It was close to 4:30 AM when I overheard the medic telling Gail that I had suffered a massive stroke, but I couldn't speak or acknowledge the news. Gail left the room to tell friends and family, and that's all I know.

I didn't experience any of the typical signs or symptoms before having my stroke. It came on fast, without warning. . . . Apparently, the bike fall at the race months before caused a tear in the skin near my left carotid artery. The skin "flapped" over the artery, causing a clot and closing off the flow of blood to the brain, resulting in a much-delayed cerebral hemorrhage. I was given blood thinners to break up the clot, but it never dissolved. The blood found another artery to take over the flow to the brain. As it turns out, I still have the clot thirteen years later.

I was paralyzed on my right side, from head to toe, and I was right-handed, so it was a total shock. I could not speak or understand anyone very well. I thought I was in a dream and would wake up soon, but unfortunately it was real! The nurses talked about me like I wasn't there, and I heard them say, "He used to be a very good athlete. Poor guy, he won't be able to do anything after this." I was lying there, unable to respond, and I was crushed.

I spent three-and-a-half weeks in the hospital without an ounce of PT, ST, or OT before being sent to a rehab center. I left the hospital in almost the same shape as when I arrived. My right hand and leg could lie flat—unlike now—but I could not move my fingers or toes, and I had no control over my limbs. They started me on OT, ST, and PT, but improvement was very slow in coming. They showed me pictures of a gorilla in a tree, and I knew what it was, but I couldn't speak or describe what I saw. I couldn't even remember my kids' names. I said to myself, "Oh my God, this is very bad." I cried a lot. They'd wheel me down to the gym and work on my leg and arm. I tried to move a ball and couldn't even nudge it. In time I could walk a bit, but I just dragged my right leg. I refused to use a walker or aids because I was in complete denial of my condition.

I spent two months there and then another ten months doing outpatient therapy. They taught me all the skills I needed to function at home: cooking, washing, even driving. They would load about six stroke patients into a van and take us to the grocery store to practice shopping. We had a list of veggies and such. It was like a sideshow as we stumbled out of the van with our various degrees of disability; quite funny, really. We had to add up the prices and budget our money, but it was almost impossible to do.

Toward the end of my inpatient rehab I was able to go home on weekends. I usually got a ride from Gail or my parents, but did walk the two-kilometer distance on occasion. I'd drag my affected leg from lamppost to lamppost. I was an athlete and a well-known face in my hometown, but few people wanted to encounter me as I walked down the street. My right arm was curled, my face was contorted, and I dragged my leg something awful, so I was scary looking. I watched people I knew actually cross the street to avoid me.

My daughters, who were eight, ten, fourteen, and sixteen at the time, came to see me at the rehab center, which was rough. I was half shut down, and in their eyes I probably looked dead. They took one look and said, "That's not my dad." It was very scary and sad for them. I felt terrible about it.

I left rehab after two months. I could drag my right leg and walk without an aid. My right arm and hand, which could lie flat before, were now curled and contorted. People could understand a few words, but I mostly mumbled. When I tried to speak in sentences I would mix up the order and say the second sentence before the first. My face was still paralyzed and drooped, and I could hardly smile, which I guess was somewhat lucky since I didn't have much to smile about. My vision was improving, but I still couldn't read.

Before my stroke we were raising four girls and getting on, you know? We were both very busy. Besides my job as a physical education teacher, Gail and I had a successful clothing design business, with Gail as the driving design force. She was stressed-out from the work and from raising kids, so I told her that I would take the next three months off work to run the girls around town and be the house-husband. The very next night I had the stroke.

During my time in the hospital and rehab, my wife and I divorced. We did do counseling, individually and as a couple, but our connection was no longer there. I had no choice but to leave the house. I remember hobbling to one of the stores we owned in town and moving into the back. I never returned to my home. . . . My daughters came to see me, and it was very sad for them and for me. Through all of the trials and tribulations, they have grown up to be fine young women. Gail brought some of my belongings to the store that I was now calling home. I had set up a kitchen and living space with utensils and a TV.

I had won the Wild Trek twice, done a fourteen-day canoe trip around the southwest coast of Tasmania in horrendous conditions, and competed in endurance cycling events. . . . No longer able to work out or race, I didn't handle the depression very well. I holed up in the apartment and smoked pot. I did that for months. That was my way of handling the stress and depression. But I was a competitor and, ultimately, a survivor. After a few months, I realized that the only way out of this predicament was to try to go back to what I knew, which was the world of fitness. I knew some of the players from the Australian Rules football team, which is very popular in Australia, and I was offered a job as Fitness Coordinator for a team called St.

Kilda. I designed a regimen specifically for them. For the off-season I recommended a collection of routines that involved resistance training in the swimming pool, beach running, cycling, boxing—all aerobic stuff to keep them in shape for the season. I worked with them for a little over a year. They went on to the Australian Rules Football Grand Final that year.

Most of the rehab I had was focused on teaching me to function in society: speaking, spelling, writing (with my left hand), adding numbers. That was all the mental stuff. Physically, I worked very hard in PT and in the gym. I used my drive and physical strength to bring myself back from my steep fall from grace. I used a Versa Climber® to help strengthen my bad leg. It's a machine that allows me to climb stairs and control the speed as the stairs revolve. I worked this machine to death. I walk on the treadmill, but can't run. I lift weights and walk and ride my bike continuously around a large block, and I do "spinning" on a stationary bike. I also unfurl my left hand and wrap it around a pull-up bar to stretch and lengthen my weaker arm. I've done some swimming, but intend to really dig into it this year.

There was no insurance for bike accidents, which caused some financial hardship for me. A friend convinced me to start doing speaking gigs to share my experience and insights, even though I felt I wasn't ready. Early on, I dragged myself to Melbourne Hospital to speak to a group of stroke survivors. It was a disturbing moment when I saw all these disabled people staring at me. I told them that it took seven years to get to where I was at the time, which must have been very difficult for them to hear, given my far-from-perfect physical condition. In hindsight, my tainted mental attitude must have presented a pretty dim picture. I was still bitter and feeling sorry for myself.

I walked out of that meeting and had an epiphany of sorts. I realized that I should have been more positive and more inspiring. I should have told them, proudly, "If you work hard, you can get to my level." Instead, I probably did more harm than good. That event changed my life and helped turn me around.

It now says "Stroke Genius" on my business card. My friend is a humorist, and he came up with the term, which came from the idea that it would take a small "stroke of genius" to recover from what happened. I ran with the idea and put together a "total health" presentation that addresses stroke, cancer, prostate, PSA tests, and blood pressure—focusing on preventive care. I also talk about diet and eating healthy, mental attitude, humor, communication, and how to enjoy life, regardless of your disability or deficit.

I put together a presentation for corporate events and school groups. I spoke to a group of thirteen- and fourteen-year-old kids just recently. I told my story and explained to them what they have to do to remain healthy as they grow up. I also explained the importance of their parents hearing the same message. Then the kids go home and push their mums and dads to seek these tests. We also talk about some of life's most challenging issues, like how to communicate when a loved one falls ill. I tell the kids that they can learn how to face these situations without running away.

I clammed up in the first few years following my stroke, but I now say what I feel. It's made me more honest. As a stroke survivor, you have to go to people, because they won't come to you. The stroke made me treat people the same, regardless of their age, disability, or disposition. In the past, I would not have given many of these people the time of day. And they wouldn't have wanted to be with me if I had. My girls are so proud of me, because the message I give people hopefully helps them improve the quality of their life by avoiding many of the illnesses that can affect everyone.

Thirteen years after my stroke, dates are still challenging to remember and organize. I also have trouble adding numbers, and I read very slowly. I have to do everything with my left hand: sending email, writing checks, brushing my teeth, buttoning and zipping. I print everything with my left hand now, and my writing is almost legible.

Doctors were quick to say that I would not see much more improvement after the first year, but I have continued to improve. I've been to America a few times to work with Erik Hansen in Boulder, Colorado. He taught me about the concept of neuroplasticity, which is the ability to bring "life" and coordination back to damaged and affected areas, such as my left leg and arm. So many parts of my body that were not working are starting to come alive, and I have Erik to thank for that. I still drag my left leg, but Erik has given me the building blocks to bring the "lift and step" back to the motion of walking.

It's been a wild ride. I am grateful for much of what I have and for what I have achieved, but I would give it all back in a minute to be "normal" again. I obviously miss my sports and competitions, but I mostly agonize over the loss of the time with my girls. I used to walk, run, canoe, and camp with them, and there's so little I can do on that level now. But for all of the difficulties, my life now is continually evolving, and I have much to be thankful for that I probably took for granted before the stroke. It's amazing the lessons that sometimes present themselves out of life's most challenging situations.

Postscript: May 2011

I am sorry to report that John passed away of a heart attack in February of 2011, during vacation at Flinders in Victoria. His oldest daughter, Jasna, had this to say:

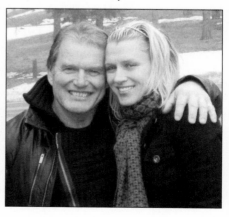

I read the interview Steve did with my dad months after his passing. It felt like a gift or message from dad, with all the answers and thoughts I never got to ask of him directly. I found it very hard to read,

because I knew what a struggle daily life was for him. His honesty reminded me of how much we take for granted. He was always working to be better. It made me very proud to see how he evolved, to see how brave and heroic he was while trying to overcome such a trauma.

After the stroke, my dad was forced to live in the moment rather than the past, every day. He inspired more people than he could imagine just by getting on with his life. I am grateful that the stroke did not take him straight away, and for giving us fifteen years to learn to love unconditionally, to focus on what life is really about. I got to know dad on a deeper, more spiritual level, and learned that we are more than just our bodies. I know that even with his passing, he will continue to serve as an inspiration. He was truly a legendary man, and he is madly missed.

KATHY & BEN

KATHY

Kathy was a twenty-four-year-old scientist with a Master's degree, employed at her first real job, when she had her strokes. The first one caused paralysis on the right side, and the second caused paralysis on the left side; both also did considerable cognitive damage. It is a fascinating story about strength, patience, and perseverance. Kathy is an energetic and alert young woman, and the second woman I've interviewed to have suffered a stroke while under the age of twenty-five.

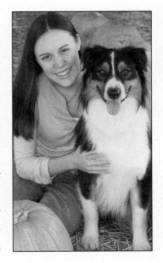

I had a TIA of sorts, though my symptoms didn't resolve within twenty-four hours the way they do with most TIAs. I woke up with symptoms one morning, about three weeks before the big one. But I knew nothing about stroke, and had no idea what was going on.

I had facial paralysis, and my husband said, "Can you fix your face?" I answered, "No, what's wrong with it?"

"It's lopsided."

I was like, "No it's not." So I went to a mirror and said, "You're right, it is!" I didn't know why, and we couldn't do anything about it, so we just ignored it.

I didn't think there was anything *too* weird going on, not yet. But then my personality changed. Ben is a computer scientist, and he works from home. I needed some programming help and asked him a technical question. He gave me an hour-long answer that I normally would have stopped after five minutes. This time, though, I just sat there listening. He thought that was strange.

Then we took a bus to a football game in town, my face still drooping. We got off the bus and he said, "Where's the stadium from here?" I said, "It's this way," which he challenged, pointing in the opposite direction. I'm a geologist by training, and I collect maps and read them for fun, so it was very bizarre that my sense of direction was so far off.

Lastly, we were supposed to meet some friends at a pizza place, but they told me that I'd written them an email the night before—which I denied—telling them that the place had burned down. When we got home, I checked my email and found I had, in fact, written that exact thing. At that point my husband said, "It sounds like you've had a stroke."

I said that couldn't be, that I must just be going crazy. My face returned to normal in three days, and my mind bounced back as well, so it left no lasting impression.

I was sitting at my desk at the National Geophysical Data Center (NGDC) when my right side completely shut down. I could speak, but it was garbled. A woman in my office asked for my husband's phone number, but I couldn't remember it. That's when they called the ambulance.

They did a CT scan at the hospital, which revealed an "old" lesion or clot from my recent TIA, which I'd forgotten about, but could now understand was linked. So I wasn't nuts, I'd actually had a stroke. The personality change from my TIA weeks earlier, which made me patient enough to listen to my husband go on about Java Script, had overtaken me again, but to a much higher degree. I was fascinated by the dye they used in the CT, flabbergasted that the service was so fast . . . everyone was doing a great job. But when they took me down for the MRI, I snapped. The paralysis was oscillating, so I'd be paralyzed for ten minutes and then fine for ten, and I just got really sad. I was having some very strange mood swings.

The MRI revealed that I'd had a stroke that hit my basal ganglia, which is unusual. That's the part of the brain that controls handwriting and such—the same place that's impaired in people with Parkinson's. I was very lucky because most of my paralysis resolved itself in a few days.

I left the hospital not knowing the cause of the stroke, but I was too fatigued to care. I was also in denial. I could walk and talk, but had some minor aphasia. My mom came to stay with me for a week or so. I did have some problems with my right hand and could not write by hand. I type 120 words per minute, so I turned to typing exclusively. I was home, and mostly bored, for six weeks.

I went back to work, but I was extremely fatigued. On my first day back I chaired a meeting about some new software, and I had to take notes. That was a disaster. I was always a strong speaker and had no problems with a crowded room, but at this point I couldn't get the words from my brain to my mouth—which is typical of aphasia. I'm in this meeting and I'm asking, "So, what can your software do for us?" But I couldn't remember the word *software,* and I pretty much lost it right there. I was totally exhausted, which was part of the reason I could not remember the word.

It's hard to recognize mental fatigue. The tendency is to push through it until you're completely physically fatigued, at which point you just crash. I am better at recognizing it now, but when I "hit the wall" I just want to check out for a while. That day I was nervous and stressed out over the presentation because of my aphasia, and stress exacerbates the condition, so it was a Catch-22. I left that position after three months.

I was in a yoga class when I had my second stroke. I noticed some people giving me strange looks, so I'm guessing that my face had started drooping. I left class and drove the short distance to my house. My vision began to blur while I was driving, and I actually missed my driveway. I was very tired and just wanted to go to sleep. I really didn't know that I was having a stroke, which is interesting because all the signs were there; luckily, Ben knew right away.

At the hospital they did an MRI, which showed that the stroke had hit my right basal ganglia. (The first stroke hit the left basal ganglia.) I spent three days in the Neuro-Ortho ward. Ben asked me some easy math questions, as I am a math whiz—yet I couldn't add twenty plus nineteen, and I couldn't tell him the cube root of a thousand, which I normally could've answered in a snap. Not only could I not give him the right answer, but it didn't bother me at all—which is really scary!

The second time I left the hospital I could walk on my own and my vision was better, but I couldn't speak very well, and my cognitive ability was in the toilet. I waited a month before trying to drive, and then had two minor accidents shortly after starting. I only hit stationary objects, so no one was hurt, but Ben suggested that I stop driving. I waited six months before trying again and have been doing well ever since.

About six weeks after the second stroke, we went on a short vacation to Las Vegas. I had never been there. I had had some bouts with up-and-down emotions over the past few weeks, where something sad would occur that made me want to cry, but instead I would laugh. They call this "emotional lability." Las Vegas can tax the emotions of even a healthy person; it was all too stimulating for me, and I started crying. At that moment, I became acutely aware of how depressed I was, and I went downhill from there. I had been taking Adderall, which is a medication for Attention Deficit Disorder (ADD), to help me get back my energy, but it had stopped working. I became extremely fatigued and petered out very early every night. The basal ganglia is the sleep center of the brain, and mine was out of whack. Back at home, Ben took me to the doctor and told her that I had cried fourteen times the day before. She prescribed Zoloft, and I was better in three days.

I had no job to go back to, so I took a part-time position teaching math at the Sylvan Learning Center. That was about a year after my stroke. . . . It was over-stimulating, and I felt that I was failing, so I left after about eight months. It did, however, help to prepare me for my next position, teaching middle school math part-time at a private school. It feels like my first permanent job, and it's been very rewarding.

I began a series of tests with a new medical team. They suspected that I had a hole in my heart, which is a relatively common cause of stroke among young people. The test results, however, were negative. I then went to a neurologist who performed a test called a transcranial Doppler (TCD). They injected my blood with micro-bubbles in an IV to see if any bubbles got to my brain. That was clearly positive; it showed that I had a big hole in my heart. I had a second TEE to confirm it. This time I was not sedated so I could perform a Valsalva maneuver to put pressure on the heart to open up the hole. They hoped to track the blood flow and find the hole when I forcibly exhaled against a closed airway. It was extremely painful.

They found the hole between my left and right ventricle, and performed a PFO (patent foramen ovale) repair. The doctors put in a latch-type thing called an occluder that blocks the hole. The heart tissue eventually grows over the device during the healing process.

My cognitive ability is still coming back, and I hope it will be completely restored some day. My memory is at about 30 percent capacity, but my math skills are back to normal, which is a good thing since I'm a scientist! I am teaching part-time, which is all I can do because of my energy level and fatigue. My handwriting is still very poor. When I try to write, the letters start out perfectly shaped for the first word, but quickly degrade into microscopic-sized print by the third word, which is common with Parkinson's sufferers. I do use the whiteboard at school, but I focus very hard and write very slowly when I'm teaching.

I hike a bit, and I hope to get back on the ski slopes this year. But I am definitely less active. I am still taking Plavix, a blood thinner, and am hoping to wean myself off the Zoloft or greatly reduce the dose this coming year.

It sucks to have a stroke—but shit happens! People say that it's "fortunate" that I had a stroke when I was young so I could have time to recover and get on with my life, but for me it was very frustrating because I didn't have a career that I could go back to. I was just getting started. I used to be very good at public speaking and had actually won contests, and I'm terrible at it now—I forget what to say.

Postscript: May 2011

I gave birth to a daughter, Norah Lynn Brantley, on April 21, 2011. She's gorgeous and, as of right now, I'm surviving the late night feedings. It feels really good to finally have a job I'm good at, even if it is just nursing and diapers!

Ben

Ben is Kathy's husband of three years. He was twenty-seven when Kathy had the first of her two strokes. He's an energetic and articulate guy, with a lot of good insights for spouses of survivors.

I got a call from Kathy's co-worker, who alerted me to her condition, but she knew very few details. I was traveling and had to sit on an airplane for three hours, worrying. I fly a lot, and it was definitely the worst flight I've ever taken. When I finally got to the hospital and the nurse filled me in, it all started to make sense: her face droop, the disorientation, the uncharacteristic behavior.

I was just so relieved to see that she was alive. Half her body was paralyzed, but she was in good spirits at that time. I was proud of her for being so brave in the face of all this. I later found out that she had this peace and tranquility partly because her brain was not functioning correctly and partly because she was disassociated from what was going on. She could not conceptualize how significant the damage was, and it took her weeks to get the drift of what had transpired. It was touching to see how positive she was as it unfolded.

The single most challenging thing is that Kathy's capabilities are unpredictable. Humans are good at adapting, so as a family we have adjusted to this radical change; but we had to learn to deal with it. I can say that she has many more good days now, compared to three years ago, but there's nothing to habituate to, because there is no constant. It's very hard to know, on any given day, if Kathy will have the energy to get out of bed—or the opposite; maybe she'll have an abundance of energy. Yesterday we did seven different things, and I was worn out, but she was still going.

Kathy has her bad days, and so do I. We have our little arguments and debates, just as any married couple does, but it often comes back to this eternal conflict between us. She will say, "You can't know or understand what I've gone through." And the truth is that she's right. On one hand, I understand her stroke better than anyone else, including her doctors and therapists, and anyone else who has not lived twenty-four/ seven with a person with this type of injury. At the same time, I have not lived it, and it will always be a point of contention between us. I'm a computer guy, so I'll use this analogy: It's like two computers trying to hook up and figure out which speed to communicate at, and it's different every time. Sometimes it's almost humorous. I have gotten much better at assessing where she is and what she's feeling, but I can still be wrong and completely miss her intention.

There's also a significant positive that's come out of this: The stroke has made Kathy a bit less obsessive-compulsive about things, which is great. She's a little more laid-back and more empathetic toward others; there's a sense of calm acceptance now about the world and her place in it, which she didn't have before. And in many ways, we've grown closer in the face of adversity. It's like going to war against a third party; we are united in that battle.

I think she remembers how she was before the stroke, but she tries to minimize her memory of that. She went through a classic case of denial and grief, slowly coming to acceptance over a two-year period. Once she got to that place, things got a lot better, a lot faster. She doesn't talk much about how it was before or about what she can't do now, which I think is good.

One of her frustrations and challenges has been to find ways to be a meaningful part of society, given her limitations. It took her a while to get her finger into handholds and start climbing again. I think she's really made some strides there, and that's gone a long way to increasing her comfort. She shows a real willingness to keep fighting. She doesn't voice much dissatisfaction and seems to have a "glass half-full" mentality.

My advice to the spouses or partners of stroke survivors: First of all, it's going to be a long, multi-year journey, during which everything will be up in the air. The survivor will be experiencing new challenges and adapting a plethora of coping mechanisms, many of which are not going to be much fun for anyone. There has to be a sense of patience and a willingness to be open and giving so the injured person has time to turn himself or herself around and to heal.

The first six months for us were a bit forgiving, because Kathy was partially in denial and somewhat mellowed by her brain injury. The period between six and eighteen months was brutal, because she had healed enough to come to terms with the reality and enormity of her condition. That was a very rough time. During this period, it's important for the healthy spouse to find ways to blow off steam, maybe by playing sports or pursuing other hobbies. I took short trips to play poker with friends so I could be completely disconnected from Kathy and my role as caregiver. I did that every three or four months. We had a good support team in both of our parents, who were glad to visit and spend time with Kathy.

Kathy and I love to debate and discuss, which is fun and stimulating for both of us, and Kathy still has that intellectual ability. Her battery is small though, so we've had to learn to recognize and then seize the right time for these debates. But she can still bring it on! Sometimes she will let her battery run down and choose *not* to joust, which is fine with me, because I know she has the ability. When her battery is full, then we go at it. The relationship changes hour by hour, which is actually kind of nice. I like the variety.

Having said that, it's different when we're out in a social setting. She loses energy pretty fast with all the stimulation.

She knows that her personality changes when she becomes fatigued, but she can't do anything about it, and it does skew other peoples' perceptions of her. It's hard for me to see her like that, so I have to watch closely and take care of her.

When we're home together, I see all these new and interesting parts of her personality that I didn't know were there. The stroke has helped her evolve and branch out in other ways. She's still beautiful and funny, and I love to be with her. We are still soulmates; nothing has changed.

DAN & CHRIS

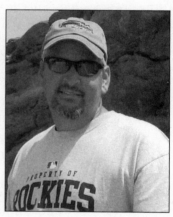

Dan was forty-four when he had his stroke two years ago. He's a big guy who hikes and snowboards—healthy and full of life. His wife, Chris, is a nurse, so she knows something about stroke.

DAN

I was driving alone, talking to a client on the phone. I wasn't feeling right, so I got off the phone and started talking to myself while I looked in the mirror. I could tell that I wasn't speaking correctly and that my face was drooping on the left side. About a minute later, my left arm went numb and it kept falling off the steering wheel. My thinking was that I had to get off at the next exit. I was *certain* there was a hospital near there, but in fact I was just disoriented; there was *no* hospital.

Luckily I was wearing an earpiece and I have pictures of my family members on my phone, so I pressed the picture of my wife and it dialed her at work. I said, "I can't talk and my left side is paralyzed."

She said, "What are you doing right now?"

"I'm driving." I had the car on cruise control and was doing 65 or 70. I kept veering off both sides of the road, knocking down reflectors and speed limit signs. My wife said, "I don't care where you are, stop now!" Her boss kept talking to me while she called an ambulance. A number of people had already called the police to report my erratic driving. A state trooper pulled up, came to my door, and asked if I'd been drinking. I said, "No, I think I'm having a stroke."

After the state trooper left to call for backup, a woman came over to me. She heard me talking on the phone and saw the tears in my eyes, and she asked if I was talking to my wife.

She said, "I'm Donna. D-O-N-N-A," which I thought was kind of strange at the time. "I've been following you for miles." She took the phone and started talking to my wife, repeating what she'd told me. She was instrumental in keeping me together. She even came to the hospital. I saw her in the ER and I said, "D-O-N-N-A,"—so I did recognize her. She stayed with me until my wife came. She asked if she could pray with me. She was my guardian angel.

In the ER, the neurologist confirmed that I was having a stroke, and that's when I first heard about tissue plasminogen activator (TPA). She told me it was a "clot buster" and said, "You fit the bill to have it: right age, good cholesterol, good general health." And I'll never forget the next part. She said, "It works on eighty percent of people, but six percent of peoples' brains bleed out, and they die."

I remember thinking, *This is a heck of a decision*. I was trying to figure it out. *So there's an 80 percent chance I'll live?* I couldn't do the odds right.

Finally, I asked her what *she* would do, and she said that I was at a low risk, so I agreed to get the TPA. The next morning the clot had dissolved and the swelling had gone down.

I spent three days in the ICU before being transferred to a rehab center, where I spent six days.

I had some sense of the severity of my situation when I was in the ER, but I *really* understood it once I was in the ICU. I couldn't feel my left leg or arm, and I couldn't move them, either. I remember thinking how lucky I was to be right-handed. I couldn't speak that well because half of my vocal cords had been affected, and I couldn't swallow solid foods for about five days.

I was very positive while I was in rehab. I made a decision early on that I would do whatever it took to get better. But I was scared, because they never give you a direct answer about how long recovery will take or how much everything will cost, so you never know. Everyone kept saying to work hard, so that's what I did.

Of course they wheel you to the door on your last day, but I could have walked out, as shaky as I was. My left arm and face were still limp. I couldn't leave until I passed a series of tests. I had to be able to brush my teeth and cook some simple meals on the stove. I had to take a trip to the grocery store and select items from a shopping list of foods that I don't normally buy. I could read the list, but identifying the foods and the labels was very frustrating because my brain couldn't compute the information. That's when I realized that my physical progress was way ahead of my cognitive progress. It was dizzying.

I slept a lot my first few days at home. I was very happy to be there and felt a tremendous amount of relief. Even though I was not the same person as the day I left for work the day of my stroke, it was a monumental step in my recovery. My wife went back to work full-time. I did some chores as best I could, but mostly laid around and watched TV. When I watched a funny show, I'd laugh and laugh; it was a huge stress relief. I didn't want to go out and didn't feel much like seeing visitors. I felt very self-conscious about eating in front of people because I was still drooling out of the left side of my mouth, which my wife would have to wipe for me. It was very embarrassing. She was still wiping my mouth a year later.

It took about three months for my cognitive improvement to start kicking in, but I had learned enough about my condition to rely on the safety steps I'd put in place; I made notes and lists, and I repeated important things. I started ordering books and reading about stroke. I read *My Year Off* and a book called *Twenty Minutes in Heaven, Twenty Minutes in Hell.* I also read a number of books on positive thinking.

Therapists came to my house for OT and PT twice a week for about four weeks. I followed that with eight weeks of outpatient PT at a medical facility. I also had some massage. After sixty days I maxed out the outpatient visits covered by insurance, and a week later I hired a personal trainer. When I started with the trainer, all I could do was walk on the treadmill. I couldn't lift my left arm above my shoulder. My hand functionality was at about 25 percent. We did a lot of work with Thera-bands and some very light weights. Even though I could walk, my balance was still wanting, so we committed lots of time to that.

I was an avid golfer, which was a big motivator to get better. I started attending a stroke support group for golfers. We all played one-handed, with our good hand. The teacher was a pro before his stroke. He told me that his last round before the stroke was a sixty-seven, and his best score since the stroke was one hundred twenty-nine. He had braces on his leg and arm, which was very depressing to me, but he also said that the one hundred twenty-nine was sweeter than the sixty-seven.

I went through bouts of depression. In the beginning, OT and PT went well and improvement came fast. Then I hit a wall, and it started to affect my spirit and my energy. I went to the doctor and said, "I'm not having any kind of suicidal thoughts, but I am really feeling down." She prescribed

Celexa, an antidepressant, and it took the edge off. I went off it after a while, but went back on a low maintenance dose. I never wanted to pity myself or feel like a victim.

I started driving again after three months, which was too early. I needed to drive in order to get to work and to see clients, but I wasn't as alert or as aware as I should have been. The biggest thing I noticed was that I wasn't always sure that red meant stop! I never drove at night, and still don't. The lights swirl and make me uneasy.

I'm not concerned about having another stroke. I did have a clot in my heart, and it did go to my brain, but I had no cholesterol problems and no plaque. In fact, I was just tested a short time before the stroke and everything was normal. The doctor still isn't sure why I had the stroke, but he also doesn't see any reason why I should have another. I was under a lot of stress at the time, but we can't be sure that stress was the cause. The docs thought it was very unusual for someone like me, with above-average stress, to have such a quick clotting process.

Overall, I feel good. I still have low energy, but I don't nap anymore because of my schedule—though I'd love to. I will, on occasion, come home whipped at five o'clock and sleep through the night. My body still aches and I have general overall weakness. I still do two days a week with my trainer and try to get out on my own once a week, if I have the energy. For me, the physical challenges have been the hardest to accept.

I think this all happened for a reason. Perhaps it was my body telling me to slow down. I have also reestablished a relationship with God. I try to live every day to the fullest, and I appreciate everything I have. First and foremost, I just want to be positive. I am thankful for what I've gotten back and hopeful that more will come.

I believe that everything happens for a reason. You have to find the good part of why this happened to you—and that's what you are doing right now by reading this book. Finding the silver lining will help you, and it certainly helped me.

CHRIS

Chris and Dan have been married almost thirty years. She is an OB nurse and knew the signs of stroke.

When Dan called from the road, I sensed right away, based on his description, that he was having a stroke. I'm a trained nurse and accustomed to stressful situations, so I jumped into action. My first concern was to get him some help. I was concerned that he might crash or lose consciousness. It was a battle between trying to get him help and controlling my fear.

I was hoping that it was just a TIA, wondering what I was going to do with my kids, and thinking about missing work; but ultimately, just hoping that he'd be alive when I got there.

Dan wasn't in great shape when I got to the hospital. He was totally paralyzed on the left side, he was teary-eyed and emotional, and he had a hard time talking; but he knew who I was and was relieved to see me. He was scared and overwhelmed by the chaos, hoping that he could go home soon. I held his hand and tried to comfort him.

I was wondering if he'd survive and be able to walk someday. I was trying to understand why he had a stroke, because he did not have many of the typical risk factors. I watched the monitors and saw the irregular heartbeat, wondering if it was a coronary artery and if he'd have a heart attack.

I had a lot of guilt leaving him because he was so emotional, and I felt like I should have stayed. It was hard to talk to the kids, because teenagers don't look outside their little world. They couldn't really grasp the weight of something so intense and complicated. They wanted me to be home, so I was getting a little bit of anger from them. They felt that I was neglecting them. They knew that he was sick, but they just didn't understand.

I cried when he first walked in the ICU. He needed help as he shuffled, but just seeing him walk down the hall made me feel that he would make it. It was a turning point, albeit a small one, but it helped me understand what I'd have to do to prepare our house for his return.

Caring for him came naturally to me after my nursing training and raising kids. On the flip side, it was very stressful having to be responsible for 100 percent of the duties at home. I knew that Dan couldn't do anything other than just be: eat, drink, and try to heal.

It may not be the right word, but I did harbor some resentment. I had to help him in and out of bed, prepare his lunch each day, clean up after him and the kids, and fill the role of both parents, in addition to working full-time. It was hard.

And it was hard to leave him alone all day while I was at work. . . . He's left the refrigerator door open, the stove burner on, the water running in the sink . . . I had to leave for work wondering about his safety and whether he'd burn the house down. It's like leaving a toddler home alone!

At first we really thought that the physical challenges would be the hardest to deal with, because he seemed to be able to answer most questions; yet there were glimpses that he wasn't all together, which was kind of shocking. Until you have to perform, you don't really know what you've lost. So I would have to say the emotional and the cognitive challenges have been even harder. The physical stuff was easy to identify, and we would get through whatever we had to. But the fragile emotions and the depression started to show after the first month at home. The details escaped us in the first few weeks because we were so focused on survival.

Our sense of humor was one of the things that helped Dan heal and cope. We've known each other so long that he could laugh at himself and I could laugh at him, in a loving way. He'd forget things and drop stuff on the floor, and spill food and drinks down the front of his shirt like a three-year-old.

Our relationship didn't suffer much. We didn't really have those "soul mate" issues; it was more the fear of losing him, and the sadness that certain parts of him wouldn't come back. It's hard to accept that there will be things that he won't be able to do, and I lament that things will never be the same.

The biggest change in terms of our relationship is that he sleeps differently. I don't sleep well with him anymore, and we don't sleep well together. He goes into another world when he sleeps. He talks gibberish. He sits up in bed and has whole conversations and then goes back to sleep without any idea of what transpired in the middle of the night. He sleeps very heavily, so when he turns my way to try and snuggle, his whole left side is dead weight and he smothers me. It's not purposeful, but it is so different to sleep with someone who's had a stroke with physical impairments. It's like sleeping with a stranger! It's a hard reality to accept after thirty years together.

And the kids don't understand the nuances. They can't get their brains around the fact that their dad is not that same person he used to be. He looks normal to most people; he can walk, talk, drive, work, and have some drinks, so it fools you. They witness his fatigue and lack of energy, but don't really get that either. They just know that he can't always play and ski with them. If he overdoes it, he'll be knocked out for a day or two afterward.

One of the other tough things for us is living with the possibility of him suffering another stroke or heart failure, even though he's taking meds for his heart that should eliminate that concern. He just had a checkup and, for the first time, the doctor said that a virus in his heart might have been the cause of his stroke—which would make his heart more susceptible to another virus in the future.

No one ever knows what might befall them, be it a car accident or some such thing, but it is a more tangible threat when you've had a stroke and heart trouble. I'm afraid of that tangible threat. We don't call the doctor when he has bouts of numbness and other weird things, and we try not to live in fear. He's tired of being afraid, so Dan has the attitude that he'll deal with whatever comes his way. He's told me that he's living on borrowed time. He's here to get his ducks in a row and to get a few things figured out, but acknowledges that he may not be here for the long haul. That makes me sad. I want to grow old with my best friend, and I hope I get to.

Spouses of stroke survivors have to understand that watching and helping someone get better from a stroke is one of the slowest processes. That word, "resentment," is applicable because it's so hard to do all the work yourself and keep it together. It doesn't do any good to wallow in being the victim of a victim. They are what they are, and you have to resolve to be in it for the long haul and take each day as it comes. You have to treat it as an adventure in the face of circumstance. And you must retain your sense of humor and laugh about it, together.

We made the decision to simplify our lives and to keep stress at bay, and it's worked for the most part. Dan much prefers where he's at now, and is much more calm and accepting. I think it comes from adjusting to how the human brain lives with the fear of the unknown and what's going to happen next. He already beat death once, and he's glad to be here. It's all part of that peace and calm.

I wake up every day thankful to be here with him. Dan's thankful that he's here, and we both embrace the perspective that things could always be worse. We're thankful that we have each other and our children.

KELLY & ED

Kelly was thirty-three and healthy when she had her stroke. She had a new boyfriend, whom she would eventually marry. She is now thirty-seven and back at work full-time after four-and-a-half years at home.

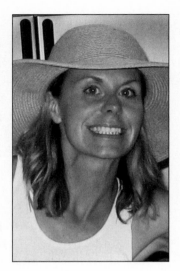

KELLY

I was in Puerto Rico with my friends for a week of sun and scuba diving. A week after our return, I was driving to work when my car stalled in the middle of an intersection. When I tried to shift gears to accelerate out of the intersection, I was disoriented and could not control the right side of my body.

I heard people honking and yelling for me to move, some of them giving me the finger as they passed. A few minutes later, two off-duty cops were at my window asking me what was going on. I told them that I couldn't get the car in gear, but that I was trying. I told them my name and age and that I was on my way to work. They asked me if I was drunk, diabetic, or on drugs, and I said I wasn't.

Then one of the cops took my cell phone and hit redial, which connected them to the last person I'd called, which was one of my girlfriends. I heard the officer telling her, "Your friend is not responding to our questions." I thought that I had been answering them the whole time, but it had actually been coming out garbled and indecipherable. When they took me out of my car, they could see that my body was shut down and quickly realized that I was having a stroke. The next thing I knew, I was in the emergency room.

As it turns out, I had suffered a cut or dissection on the left side of my carotid artery, which resulted in paralysis on my right side. The doctors presume that it occurred during my scuba-diving excursion, perhaps from ascending too quickly, but they can't be sure. The dissection could not be managed with a stent because of the size of the injury, so they put me on a blood thinner and watched me closely in the ICU for eleven days. Since they could not put in a stent to open and revive the artery, it just shut down. People can survive with just one carotid artery. However, with only one, my other vessels went into overdrive to supplement the blood flow to the brain.

When I came to, my face was numb and tingly, my right side vision was all but gone, and I could only speak four words: "toe," "stupid," "fuck," and "shit." I'd try to say, "Hi," but I would say "fuck" instead. I knew it was wrong, but that's what came out. I have no idea why it was those four words, but it was terribly embarrassing! I knew I was in bad shape and that this would be a lifelong recovery, but I also knew that I would beat this thing.

My dad and brother were notified, and they came running. Ed— my boyfriend of six weeks at the time— came too, which is how he met my family for the first time! Fortunately I am left-handed and could eke out a few letters on a pad of paper. I wrote the word "Go" and showed it to Ed, meaning, "I'm in no shape to date, so you should just move on." Thankfully he declined and stood by me. He is truly an angel. We dated for a year and a half and have now been married for two years.

I spent ten days in the ICU and then had four weeks of in-patient rehab. I was floored by the extent of my disabilities, but gave it my all during speech therapy and workouts in physical therapy. When I left the rehab hospital I could speak simple sentences, but would often leave out words.

… All in all, I did four weeks of in-patient rehab and then a full year of outpatient. The last six months were mostly devoted to speech and occupational therapy, because my physical coordination came back faster. I still have aphasia, and I still have trouble with multi-syllabic words, but I am doing home therapy and it is getting better.

My mom had died four months before my stroke and I was still reeling from that, so it was a very tough time for me. I lived alone, so my father, who is self-employed, moved in with me for six months to help with the cooking, drive me to three hours of rehab every day, and to provide emotional support. My first weeks at home were fragile and very foreign. I was excited to be home, but physical and speech therapy were extremely exhausting, so I took long naps every day. My friends would come over and take walks with me. I cried daily because I had always been a very independent person and now I couldn't even pour a cup of coffee. I went through a period of asking, "Why me?" and it took time to get past that. Still, I did say to myself at the end of each day that this is a blessing; I am still living.

I did acupuncture, which I think helped my speech and my vision. . . . I also took antioxidants, chelated minerals, Omega 3s, B12, C, and extra E. I was diligent about doing therapy at home. I would hold things in my right hand and favor it over my healthier left hand in order to continue strengthening it. I loved the challenge of sitting and balancing on a big exercise ball during my rehab sessions. Running was an addiction before my stroke and became a favorite therapy afterward. Nine months after my stroke, I ran a half-marathon for the National Stroke Association. I ran thirteen miles in two hours, fourteen minutes and raised over $15,000 for the organization.

I worked very hard on my verbal skills because they were lagging behind my physical improvements. I'd go to lunch with friends, and it would be very hard for me to keep up with the conversation. My friends supported me, and I encouraged them, so they'd be comfortable with my disabilities.

I told them it was perfectly fine to "step on my words" in order to help with my pausing and fluency issues. Some of them actually read books about stroke to better understand my condition.

Going back to working full-time after four-and-a-half years out of the workplace is exhausting, and I find it hard to muster the energy to do the therapy every day. In some ways, my work is now my therapy. I had a lot of energy before my stroke, so I'd run and ride after work. I love exercise, but I'm now too fatigued to do much physical activity. I didn't think I would ever be able to work a forty-hour week, but my employers have been very good at working with me. I still can't read or type at my pre-stroke level, but they are getting better all the time.

In my daily life I don't think about having another stroke, but my husband and I do want to have a family. Carrying a baby puts a lot of pressure on the vascular system, and I'm scared that I might have another stroke during pregnancy or delivery. We'll start researching this more seriously down the road, but we are both okay with adoption if it comes to that.

It's a constant battle. If I don't write things down, I will forget them. I may remember something a week later, or it may just be lost in space. I've lost my keys, I've lost my cell phone, I've misplaced my purse at least fifteen times . . . I left my purse on a ferry once, and I just stood on the pier screaming at the boat to come back.

I am much more compassionate and patient now. I believe that the stroke was fate. I used to feel that I had something to prove to people, but now know I don't have to prove anything to anyone. My last four-and-a-half years were totally focused on me, which I was not used to. Before my stroke, I needed to know that everything was okay with family and friends, and then I'd deal with me. But now I say, "This is my life, and I have to take care of myself first in order to help others."

Postscript: May 2011

I am different because of my stroke. Little successes, like saying multi-syllabic words without difficulty, were huge accomplishments. A few years ago, I could muster only enough energy to work part-time. I now work full-time. My company has been very supportive, which has helped me regain my courage and confidence.

Success is not final and failure is not fatal. Celebrate the little successes and if you fail, it is not the end. There is always a new opportunity waiting. I wish everybody could experience stroke for just a day, to better understand. They would appreciate every second of life—even the bad moments. It would change them forever. It did for me, and I'm blessed for that.

ED

Ed had been dating Kelly for two months at the time of her stroke and went on to marry her. He's now thirty-eight years old.

I was in shock when I saw Kelly in the ICU. My prevailing thought was that stroke was for old people. She couldn't speak but a few words, and two of them were profane. I could see the shock in her eyes, but I also saw the Kelly I knew. I had a sense of pragmatic reality: This is what it is, let's see what it becomes. It's one of those adventures that you go through. It hit me that night. I remember walking out of the hospital feeling like, "Holy shit, what are the ramifications of this?"

But I said to myself, "I'm not just going to say, 'See you later.'" That's not my style. Some of my friends intimated that since it was a new relationship I still had time to jump ship, but I had no intention of doing such a thing. She was still the same person to me, and she could still say a lot with her eyes.

I was there for her, and I was part of the healing process. I helped with whatever needed to be done. We spent time together when we could, whether we were hiking or venturing out for our first dinner. It was a gradual process, and a constant evolution. I could see her coming back, forging new neural pathways and finding ways to communicate. Her father went home after about nine months, and I moved in.

We were very close when we were dating before the stroke. It was a great two months. But 99 percent of the time I've known her has been post-stroke, and some traits take years to reveal themselves. She sure talks a lot less! When we were dating, she was very outgoing that way. But it's still the same person behind the conversation, and more thought goes into what she's saying now. If she's tired, she's not going to waste energy on mundane chitchat.

The most important advice I have for the families and loved ones of stroke survivors is that you have to wait and see, because the person you love is still there. Yes, they're different, but people change and evolve regardless of whether or not they've suffered a stroke. Stroke survivors are going to teach you patience, because they can't function as they did before. Kelly taught me those things early on because we couldn't communicate at the same pace. Things had to slow down a bit, which was great in some ways but frustrating in others. But, is it worth stressing because you can't get out the door in five minutes or you can't always reach a conclusion in ten seconds? It's about patience, and giving the person the time and respect to express themselves.

We experienced some discomforting stuff in the beginning. When she would speak in social situations, some people could not understand what she was saying. They were trying to be funny by asking if she was from Sweden or if she was drunk, but it was hurtful. After the fifth time, she would say, "Hey, I had a stroke! Go fuck yourself!" They would be mortified. We would laugh about it, but it was hard to go through.

Still, I've seen continued improvement. Every six months or so she will plateau, and then all of a sudden something radical and new reveals itself, whether it's sudden gains in her speech or something physical. We still bike and ski and hike and do all the things that were a part of our lives before the stroke. She may not perform at the same level, but she still enjoys the same activities and experiences.

Kelly can be a little forgetful, but on a day-to-day basis it's a lot of small stuff. . . . I'm more concerned about the house or car doors being locked; I will remind her about that with some regularity. She gets a bit irked at times because I keep reminding her, but I'm also a bit of a space cadet. She'll tell me something that I'll forget, and I'll tell her she never told me, so it goes both ways. We'll usually laugh about it.

If we know that something has the potential to be problematic, we will openly say, "What do we have to do to make this work?" She has learned to accept the flow of chaos, deal with what she can, and worry less about that which she can't control. There is a calmness in not having to sweat some of the details, but she is still frustrated by the occasional cognitive confusion and having to let things go.

I like to think she is satisfied with life, and I know that she is genuinely happy the majority of the time. That being said, she is still very aware of the changes. Had the stroke not occurred, we'd probably already have kids. On the career front, she had a great job in the software field that she can no longer do. Financially, she had been earning two and a half times more than what she currently earns. It's been hard to make the transition to what she has now, but she's dealt with it. She has responded by finding new and available opportunities—and her life continues.

The biggest challenges are the most rewarding. You can choose to take the easy route, or you can stay the course and deal with it as you go. I think Kelly said it very poetically, that "you have to remind yourself of what you have." And from my perspective, it is your experiences—both good and bad—and how you respond to them that make up this thing called life.

Tim & Sue

Tim was fifty-three when he had his stroke. He had retired a few years prior, gradu- ated from ministry school, and was enjoy- ing life. Like Marvel and Karen, his stroke may have been a result of a whiplash-type injury. He is fifty-five today.

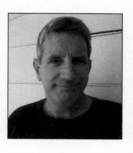

Our family was in Bend, Oregon, on vacation. I was jog- ging up a trail along the Deschutes River when I tripped over an exposed root. I fell, but I jumped back up. I got a sudden neck ache and a little headache from the jolt, but I still ran an- other mile. After the run, the headache got so bad that I went to the hospital. They treated me for a migraine. My head still hurt, so I didn't sleep much that night.

Alone the next morning, I felt a tingling sensation come over my head and the whole right side of my body. It eventu- ally hit both sides; my right side was numb, and my left side completely shut down. I couldn't stand and could only move my head and neck. My wife returned about ten minutes later and called 911. I was in a coma for two weeks and woke up with no memory beyond the ambulance ride.

I had suffered an arterial dissection in my brain, which is a tear in the blood vessels. Besides suffering pneumonia while in the coma (which I contracted twice more over the next six months), they had also performed a tracheotomy to help me breathe and a craniotomy, where they removed a two-inch by four-inch part of the skull to gain access to the tear and ad- dress the swelling in my brain.

I'm not sure what caused the stroke. My vessels may have been hardened and brittle from the twenty years I smoked cigarettes. However, I read a report that said that blood vessels can heal after five years, and I had quit smoking almost twenty years before. So while I can't be sure, I think that the fall and the whiplash was the cause.

I don't remember much about the time right after waking from my coma. I could only open one eye. I knew that I was in a hospital, but had no idea what had happened to me. I was very tired. I was in the ICU for about a month, and then in the hospital another two weeks. They did some PT, using machines to help me sit up and stand. This part felt really good after being on my back in a bed for five weeks.

Soon my face was back to normal, and my vision was temporarily better than before. My speech was badly slurred, and I spoke very slowly. My right side was numb, but working—I am right-handed, thank God. My left arm and leg kind of worked, but I had no control and no strength in my limbs.

I was pretty immobile when I left the hospital after six weeks. I was improving, but I still had a tube in my throat and one in my stomach and couldn't really speak. I was also still recovering from the aftereffects of pneumonia. I checked out of the hospital in Oregon, and my wife and I were flown home. I then spent four-and-a-half months in a hospital and another month in a nursing home.

The nursing home was terrible. I was nauseous and vomiting from the medications, and I lost fifty pounds during my stay. They did very little physical therapy, and I spent most of my time in bed or being pushed in a wheelchair. I tried to get my arms to move the wheels on the chair, but I was weak and not very good at it. I could not get the wheelchair into the bathroom, so they put me in a diaper and left me alone—which was very humiliating. I needed complete assistance. At my wife's request, I was taken off most of my meds, which helped me recover a lot of my health and sanity. However, after getting off the meds, I became aware of the people around me, most of whom were sick and screaming. I couldn't wait to get out of there.

My first few days at home were pretty rough. . . . I just sat around most of the time. I'd had twenty-four-hour care at the hospital, and I was demanding. My wife took a year off from teaching to take care of me, and I caused a lot of stress for her and my two children.

I think Sue and the kids would say that I was a demanding person before the stroke. I was stressed from work and I unloaded on them. Now, I cry when anything touches my heart. Not so much with movies and such, but when something bad happens to my family or one of my friends. The same is true when people reach out to help me.

I think the total treatment cost was about three million dollars. We were down to our last dollar. My wife had stopped working so that she could care for me, which contributed to our situation. We are fine now, but it was pretty tight for a while.

I sleep well, but I am still fatigued and wake up tired. I take an hour nap almost every day. My left side is still partially messed up. I can walk fairly well, unassisted, but my balance is bad. I walk a mile most days and up to four miles on some days. My right side is still "skin-deep" numb, but I can shower and shave and take almost complete care of myself. I started going to the gym about three weeks ago; I'm working my arms and doing some light pressing. I exercise three to four times a week and my energy level is getting much better.

I'm doing well cognitively. I started reading one word at a time at about four months, and I eventually got to a point at nine months where I could read and comprehend. Emotionally, I still get very teary. I was on a very light antidepressant after my stroke, while I was in the hospital. I now take an organic antidepressant, a combination of adaptogens and herbs that's supposed to help people cope with stressful conditions. It also improved my restless leg syndrome in one day. . . . I was taking about ten medicines when I left the hospital, but now only take one baby aspirin a day.

This was a hot topic in our support group. Most of the people agreed that they felt much better when they got off all the meds they were prescribed.

I think support groups are very, very important. Whether it's friends, church, or community, your support network can help explain things to caregivers and family members that you can't always articulate yourself or even recognize on your own. I go to my support group twice a month.

Personally, I have found more joy in my life since my stroke. Things are more real to me, and I appreciate life more. Spiritually, I seek God more than I used to. The people at my church stayed with me throughout. They came to visit me in the hospital so often that the guards thought I was a celebrity.

Still, I would trade having a stroke for having a heart attack in a minute. I cherish the emotional aspects, but I used to be very active, and now I'm not. I really enjoyed working with my hands, and now I can't even hold a screw. But I'm getting closer, and looking forward. I am hopeful.

SUE

Sue and Tim have been married for eighteen years. They are the parents of two teenage girls. Sue is back to teaching full-time after taking a year off from work to care for Tim.

Tim had a history of headaches. He took Tylenol a few times a week, so I was slow to realize that this was something different. When he told me that this was the worst headache he'd ever had and I took him to the hospital, he was having trouble walking. I suspected that it was more than just a headache, but really had no idea what it could be.

He walked like an elderly man. He couldn't get out of the car, so I got him a wheelchair. Then he said that he couldn't sit up, so I got him a gurney and helped him lie down. The doctor who saw him diagnosed him with a migraine. Then he threw up in the car on the ride back to my mother-in-law's place. He continued to complain about the pain even after taking the migraine medicine, but we were hoping he would be able to sleep it off.

I found him on the floor. He was totally conscious and told me to call 911. One side of his body didn't work, including his face. At the hospital they did an MRI and inserted a line into his femoral artery. They could then see the dissected artery in his neck, the blockage, and later, the bleeding.

The next day Tim could not recognize his daughter. He couldn't speak clearly, swallow, or breathe on his own. His neurologist told me that if they did not do a craniotomy, he would probably die. I told the doctor that dying isn't the worst thing that can happen to someone if they are going to end up a vegetable on life support, or spend the rest of their days in a nursing home. I told him that he had to give me some better information or some guarantee that the procedure would most likely help. He could not give me that assurance, but did say that Tim would most likely die if they didn't do something very soon.

I asked to speak with the doctor privately. I asked him if it were his wife in my husband's situation, would he do the surgery. He did not answer right away. Then he said he would choose surgery to give his wife a chance. His wife happens to be the head doctor at the hospital we were in, and in charge of rehabilitation for brain injuries.

I called our immediate family, and I called the elders in our local church and asked for their fellowship and prayer. I didn't want to make this life-and-death decision on my own. I then had the peace to give the neurologist the go-ahead to do the surgery.

Tim was very needy after coming home. In the hospital he would keep pushing his call button. Eventually the nurses told him that they couldn't keep running into his room every few minutes. He actually dove out of bed more than once and injured himself, so they got him what they call a "sitter"—a twenty-four-hour licensed vocational nurse. When he got home, he needed help about every ten minutes, very much like a newborn baby. He was only home for a few days before having to go to a nursing home because of a MRSA infection. I was sad for him, but his stay in the nursing home did help him get over needing attention every ten minutes. The second time he came home he was a lot easier to care for.

I've noticed many personality changes in Tim. First of all, his diplomacy is a thing of the past. Tim functions basically without a filter. He used to look at a situation, think it over, and then suggest or decide. Now he's very quick to answer, and it's not always the best way to go.

So, for example, Tim is quick to offer directions. Unfortunately, while his directions were correct before the stroke, he's now sometimes wrong. I have to find a way to deal with his input when it's a bit off, without hurting or offending him. We have to find ways to support him, without doing everything he wants us to do. It's a delicate balance, and very challenging.

He was somewhat difficult when he was in the hospital, and we talked about it one day. I mentioned something about divorce, which took him aback, even in his drugged condition. I told him that divorce and stroke sometimes go together, and there are reasons for that. With all the changes he was going through, it would be very appealing to not have to deal with them.

I remember he said, "You would really leave me in this condition?" I answered, "Well, if you're not going to deal with how you're affecting us and put some effort into seeing how *we* feel instead of only focusing on how *you* feel all the time, then I will have to take care of our needs somehow."

I'm not going to divorce Tim, but I did have to change the way we live together by giving him and me some space. He is my husband, I love him, and I am committed to our relationship. That's why I cannot let myself get burned out.

We have two teenage girls, one fifteen and one seventeen. It's very challenging, on many fronts, and tough on both of them. Tim used to spend a great deal of time with them. He took them places, helped with their schoolwork, and built props for their theatrical performances. They don't have that anymore.

Our older daughter was very close to her dad, and it's been especially traumatic for her. She tries to talk with him, but it's not the same. She doesn't get the support and nurturing she used to get. He tells her things, with his best intentions, but somehow it often ends up with both parties being frustrated. Girls, and most women, are accustomed to "filtered" advice. It's not that Tim's advice is bad or wrong, it's just that blunt remarks don't go over that well, especially with daughters.

Our older daughter is mature enough to recognize what's going on, but she's grieving the loss of their relationship and the way it was before. Our younger daughter is bitter and has not yet arrived at the same place as her sister. Tim tends to see the half-empty side of things. He gags, coughs loudly, and makes choking noises. Conversations with him are quite often frustrating for her. His mannerisms and propensity to be contrary aggravate her, so she tends to ignore him. We are still working on that.

There was a strain before, as there often is with young girls, but there's just so much more of it now. I do stick up for him. Even though he's abrupt and makes decisions so quickly, Tim is actually maturing and growing as a human being, and I'm very proud of him. I find him to be more genuine than I've ever known him to be. But from a kid's point of view, it's really hard to see the positive side, because the girls are subject to his decision-making process.

We don't want to be hurtful to him by ignoring his thoughts, but we are still just navigating the waters here. We have to watch over the girls, especially our youngest, so her heart doesn't get hard towards her dad, given his current challenges.

. . . We did have some of the brothers from the church come talk to us, one of whom was a doctor. He basically said that I have to find a way to be one with Tim and help the girls learn to have a proper attitude toward him, whether they agree with him or not. I can't say that I am clear about how to do that, but I did feel it was good advice, and we are working on it.

Tim works out at the gym and does a lot of physical therapy, and he talks to people from the church and from his support groups, but has not had traditional talk therapy. We could both use help along those lines.

Sleeping is different now because much of Tim's body is shut down. Cuddling is not as easy, and I feel smothered. As far as sex is concerned—and I say this for the benefit of other spouses—I know that he's still a man, with manly needs, but after we made sure that everything still worked, I had to beg off for a while. It wasn't too many months ago that I was helping him go to the bathroom, so it's hard for me to be intimate. He is willing to give me some time, because I'm just not ready yet. I feel a bit guilty about it, but I'm asking for time so I don't harbor resentment.

There is a tendency for the healthy spouse to feel more like a caregiver and parent than a wife or husband. It's unavoidable, because it's a lot of work and mostly uphill. Tim was a huge contributor around the house. On top of his regular job, he also paid the bills, took care of the yard and all the maintenance, did laundry, cooking, and dishes, and drove everywhere we went. I guess I didn't realize just how much he did until he wasn't able to do it anymore.

But I do believe that he will get better. Even though Tim is really different, I still believe that we can be happy together. We are both learning to live with his limitations. Because we are believers, we open up to each other and talk, and then we go to the Lord together. After praying, we forget about our difficulties and just go on. That is why I think we're going to be okay. We have accepted our situation; we're not in a hurry to see certain results outwardly. Our situation is *not* our main focus in life.

I think Tim used to have somewhat of an anxiety-driven existence before his stroke. I think the stroke alleviated much of his anxiety, and he has dramatically changed. There's no politics with him anymore. He is who he is. He's not worried about anything anymore.

Open up and seek help from everyone you can, especially the Lord. The many decisions, from hospital procedures to rehabilitation, are extremely hard to shoulder on your own, and we are not wired to know how to react to all of this.

KAREN & PASCO

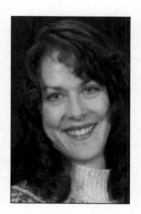

Karen is forty-seven years old. It's been nine months since she had her stroke. She still walks with a limp, and her vocal chords are still recovering, so she speaks gingerly, but she is a strong woman. Karen was finishing a PhD in social work when she had her stroke. She sang in a barbershop quartet and was making great strides as a collegiate ice skater.

KAREN

I was in a skating lesson, working on a challenging camel spin, when I fell back off my heel and onto my head. I lay there screaming in pain. I thought that I had sustained a whiplash. I did a series of massages over a three-week period to relieve the burning in my neck. It intensified during the week prior to the stroke.

After I had the stroke, I learned that I had a congenital defect in the vertebral arteries in the back of my head; the vessel on the right side is smaller than the left, and there was a tear in the lining. Over a five-week period, the blood had pooled and then clotted in the tear and closed off the artery. It might be considered a dissection.

The morning of the stroke I felt the burning again. Then the right side of my face started tingling and my arm went numb, so I knew something bad was happening. Fortunately my husband had not yet left for work. When I called Pasco, he said that my face was white as a sheet. He asked what I was feeling, but I had lost my ability to speak. I had trouble breathing, and then I blacked out.

Pasco called 911, and I was on oxygen within five minutes. They said that if I had been alone and had lain there all day I probably would have died or been seriously disabled, so I was very lucky.

When the EMT guys revived me, I had impaired vision, a bad case of hiccups, and I was retching something awful. By the time I got to the ER, my whole right side was paralyzed (I'm right-handed), and my face was completely drooped.

I spent the first six days in the hospital on heparin, with an oxygen tube in my nose. I just lay in bed. I was rarely given a shower. They combed my hair and did some minor exercises, but I was very upset that I wasn't being taught to walk. I wanted more physical therapy, but all they offered was speech therapy, which only consisted of swallowing training, though I was too nauseous to eat for the first four or five days.

By the sixth day I showed considerable improvement. I could speak a bit, though my speech was strained because my vocal chords were damaged. I could identify the people in my room and was much more aware. Other than some memory issues, I thought my mind worked well.

After a week I was well enough to be transferred to a nursing home. However, I woke the next morning complaining that my left side was feeling strange and was immediately taken *back* to the hospital. They said that the affected area was now larger. I didn't have another stroke, but the condition had spread to my left side as well. I was transferred to a rehab center, where I spent two weeks. They taught me how to walk, and I made real progress physically.

By the time I left rehab my facial droop was gone. I could walk short distances with a walker and sometimes with a cane, and my arms were mostly functional. I had severe balance problems and vertigo and could not bend over. But if I could have, I would have been able to tie my own shoes. Pasco found a cane, a walker, and a wheelchair on Craigslist, so I had everything I needed. I also was getting in-house physical therapy three times a week and speech therapy twice a week.

My parents came and took care of me. It was pretty weird and very humbling to have my seventy-something mother bathe me. Pasco and I are still kind of newlyweds, so it was a little hard on him to have my parents staying in the house. But he's self-employed and had missed a lot of work over that past month, so he couldn't stay home. He knew that I couldn't be left alone, and we couldn't afford to hire anyone, so he was thankful that my parents were there. They were a tremendous help.

I also had trouble sleeping. Because of my balance issues, I had to wake Pasco in the night to walk me to the bathroom. I had a sensation that I was falling out of bed, but never did. I was still wearing an eye patch on my right eye.

I had full insurance, which is very fortunate because the first month was over $100,000. I am paying $50 a month toward associated medical bills. I'm still very concerned because I will need hearing aids, new glasses, and more physical therapy.

I became very depressed at about two months after the stroke. At four months, I started to work on my PhD again, but between my impaired vision and my mental state, I had a rough time. When I was still hurting at six months, I began to believe that I would not make a full recovery, and I started down a very dark road. I remember thinking, "Oh, my God, maybe this is it." They told me that I should make a full recovery. But I still walked like I had cerebral palsy and still had all these pains in my face. I used to sing in a barbershop quartet and wanted to sing in a mixed group with my husband, but my voice has not come back enough to participate.

I actually started working again at about three weeks, seeing two clients at a time on a part-time basis. I have a small therapy practice, specializing in transgender issues. I got a pass from the rehab hospital, and they assigned a helper to get me to work. I used a small room in my husband's office for these early meetings. I could hardly speak, and looked horrific, but it did me good and did a lot for my clients. They were moved by my strength and drive, and were very relieved to see me there and alive. It gave me purpose.

After five months I started acupuncture twice a week. I really couldn't afford it and had to cut back to once a week, which was not a good thing, and it showed. My very sweet and caring acupuncturist reduced my fee so I could go back to twice-a-week care. Thank God for him. The acupuncture helped me become stronger, my vision has improved, and the pain in my eye went from excruciating to bearable. My balance is also better.

Shortly after my stroke, our landlord went bankrupt and we were forced to move. I could barely walk, but here I was packing and hauling boxes most of the day. Then there was the moving and unpacking and cleaning. By this point my husband was kind of done dealing with the stroke situation, and he would ask me what I did all day. He expected a lot more out of me than I could deliver. I'd say, "Honey . . . stroke!"

He didn't mean to be insensitive, but he was frustrated and traumatized by the whole thing. He almost lost me, and he was still reeling from that. He's learning that it takes me five times as long to do everything now.

I began skating when I started my PhD program. I won an adult competition about two weeks before my stroke. I was preparing for the intercollegiate national championship competition out of state with my team, which would have been that weekend. I got back on the ice three months after the stroke and rejoined the collegiate team. My doctor said that although skating is a bit riskier than most activities, I could reinjure my artery by merely climbing the stairs, so I might as well go live my life.

Progress was slow for me due to my artificial knees and the fact that I began skating as an older adult. Unfortunately, after two months of struggling with relearning to skate from scratch, the powers that be implemented a new age rule that cut me off, so I quit skating altogether. I'm finally done pouting about that and ready to go back. I will now skate in the recreational adult competitions at the beginner level again.

Despite all my physical and mental challenges, skating at any level makes me feel whole. Several people have balked at the mention of my return to the ice after my stroke, but they don't understand that one must *live* their life, not merely *wait it out* in safety, hoping that nothing bad happens.

These days, my right eye is still a bit cloudy, but it's getting better. The right side of my face tingles, and I have this itchy, cold feeling. . . . The double vision took about three weeks to resolve, but I still have two different-sized pupils, which makes reading difficult. I have trouble scanning across a page and I set my computer monitor to magnify the writing. I close an eye, squint, and tilt my head to help my vision.

My left hand is still weak, so I can't pick things up. My left side feels like a bucket of ice water, my left leg hurts, and I have neuropathy (nerve damage and reduced control). When I'm tired, my voice goes. I also have ADD. On top of my other challenges, I had knee replacements at thirty, a hysterectomy, and I'm bipolar, so I've had quite a colorful life. I've been taking Wellbutrin for my depression, but I'm on a low dose because it causes ringing in my ears. I've also gained twenty-five pounds, which has been hard mentally and physically, but I use eating as an emotional crutch. I clearly have motivational problems, but hope to persevere and finish my PhD.

As for my cognitive ability, I started playing Sudoku while I was still in the hospital. My husband got me easy games in big print, and I have continued to play them at home on the Internet. These puzzles helped me get back some skills.

I try not to dwell on the possibility of having another stroke. The doctor said that I may never have another or I may have one next week. The weakness in the artery makes it unpredictable, and the area was too small to stent. It makes me even more stubborn about doing what I want to do. My biggest fear is not necessarily about having another stroke, it's about having a stroke that leaves me completely disabled. If I do have another stroke, I hope it kills me, because I don't want to live with any more disabilities than I have now.

I'm just now coming to grips with the fact that my life has permanently changed. I feel old. At the three-month mark, when two medical people told me that I should've died, I began feeling like I may have been a little too ungrateful for all the good things in my life. There's a tenacity about me that's a bit annoying, but also inspirational. I don't give up.

Postscript: May 2011

I went back to skating with my collegiate team (even competing at nationals and winning a medal!) and graduated with my PhD in social work in August of 2010. I am currently the new Program Director for the Gender Identity Center of Colorado. Although my skating is not what it was, I still take lessons and skate a couple times a week.

PASCO

Pasco and Karen were relative newlyweds when Karen had her stroke.

I was relatively calm as I called 911, but my initial thought was that Karen was having a stroke. The EMTs arrived within five minutes. I spent the next three days wondering if she would survive. Watching her suffer like that was very disturbing. The doctors made remarks suggesting that she might never walk or speak again, and may even have to be institutionalized. In retrospect, those first days—when we were in the dark about her condition—were some of the lowest and darkest days of my life.

The doctors had ruled out a surgical procedure for the artery tear in favor of the "watch and see" method. She was taking Coumadin, and we all relaxed a bit once the clot had dissolved. After a few weeks they sent her to a nursing home with a bunch of elderly people, where she began to experience burning in her neck and face, similar to what she felt before the stroke. They sent her back to the hospital. The ER doc wanted to start all the tests over again, and I had to insist that she first read the damn records before doing any more tests. It was a nightmare. Finally they sent her to a rehab hospital, where they actually knew how to care for stroke patients properly.

It was not exactly what we had in mind for our marriage. We never dreamed that our happy lives would come to a halt over something as seemingly innocent as a fall. There were times when I needed to chill out and take thirty minutes to regroup. At times I became angry and just wanted to lash out.

Another low point came about four months later when the doctors said that she was about as good as she was going to get—and she was only at maybe sixty percent. It was at this point that she started acupuncture, which brought back much of her eyesight and voice.

Karen is adamant that the acupuncture treatments have been monumental in her recovery, and I absolutely agree with her. Besides improving her eyes and voice, it has certainly helped her emotional outlook. It helped her recover much more than sixty percent of her faculties. As a result, Karen is now probably close to ninety percent, except for her long-term physical deficits. I highly recommend it for all stroke survivors.

I always worry about her when she's out, when she's driving, when she doesn't answer the phone. The doctors told her that she could suffer another stroke because the artery is so weakened. They also said that she might not survive another stroke, and that she could suffer a stroke by simply walking up the stairs.

These thoughts are not in the forefront of my mind, but they're certainly in the back. I keep thinking that I might come home one day and find her sprawled on the floor or slumped over the steering wheel. I am haunted by the thought that I might not be there to help her, and I have to live with this every day.

I'm not crazy about Karen continuing to ice skate. Karen's attitude is that she's going to live her life. I know she's a free spirit, and I love that part of her, but falling on the ice is a lot different than walking up the stairs. I can't tell her what to do, so it's a constant worry for me. But I am proud of her strength.

It's extremely important for anybody in the hospital for an extended period to have an advocate. Even with me watching every move, there were times that we had to get the patient advocate. Workers and custodial staff walked in on Karen half dressed, without knocking, and there was a lot of inappropriate behavior by X-ray technicians and other staff. One doctor actually had the gall to say that Karen was faking her condition to get attention, and Karen was right there, lying in bed with one eye shut, unable to speak or respond. If she were faking, it would have been an Academy Award-worthy performance.

I was livid. We made sure that Karen always had family around, but having a patient advocate is a must. I couldn't always be there because of my dental practice; If I'm not at work, we're not making money. It was a huge stress having to miss appointments and cancel patients. That was another reason for us to bring in family and friends to help out.

Karen did not have any severe cognitive issues; she's still funny and still has her sense of humor. But she had a lot to accept, on many levels. She had to relearn to walk, which was traumatic for her. Karen used to be very graceful and athletic. She danced and ice-skated quite beautifully for an older woman (compared to the twenty-year-old girls in her group). She now struggles to walk and tires easily. I've had to become much more perceptive about her moods and need for rest. We both have to be aware of her blood sugar because she zones out. She gets extremely fatigued, which taxes and depresses her.

Life has definitely slowed down. Things take a lot more preparation, be it leaving the house for a movie or an appointment, or just walking down the stairs. I will stand next to her or in front of her to steady and support her. We don't walk as much as we used to because it's just too hard.

Karen's elderly parents stayed with us the first few weeks she was home from the hospital. It was very sweet of them, and it was mostly a good thing. I did go through some rough periods when her mother rearranged my underwear drawer in the dresser. I was already mentally fragile, and I felt it was a bit intrusive. However, it was great for Karen, and I think it helped her acclimate back to our home without putting additional stress on her.

Between work and extra care duty, I have sometimes been negligent when it comes to taking care of myself. I probably could have used some therapy as well. I'm just starting to work out a bit, but I have been very sedentary for most of the past year.

The most important thing is to be patient, because it's a long road. Try to be aware of the circumstances, early on, and reach out for an advocate at the hospital at the first sign of problems. Lastly, it's a life change, and the spouse will never be the same because of what they've gone through. Regardless, the partner or spouse has to be on board and supportive, even when there's nothing they can do to help. The stroke hasn't really changed our personal relationship, but we have become closer in the face of adversity.

Our relationship was a Cinderella story before the stroke. I never thought that I would find a soul mate so late in life, but I did; and then everything became distorted. I wanted to take care of Karen and watch over her for the rest of our lives, and I still do, but I never thought it would be as a result of a stroke. It's a different life and it's a shame, but I love her and will always be there for her.

DON & GRACE

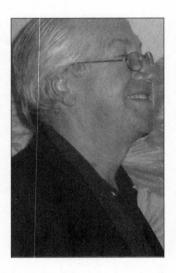

Don had his stroke at fifty-six and is now sixty. His is a colorful story, accentuated by the fact that he was aware of his high blood pressure and knew that some of his personal habits were aggravating this condition. He is a painter and an artsy guy, a college professor, and an admittedly stubborn man.

DON

I had driven my wife Grace to the airport in the morning, and I was having dinner at home with my ninety-eight-year-old mother, who lived in the front of the house. I had been drinking off and on since two o'clock that afternoon, and had probably ingested a bottle-and-a-half of wine by dinnertime. I went to my bedroom, where I promptly fell to the floor.

I tried to do a push-up and actually rolled over because my left arm was too weak to support that half of my body. I assumed that I'd had too much to drink or that I was coming down with the flu. My mother called Grace and told her that I was on a "bender" and that I didn't look or sound good. My left side remained weak, and I could see that the left side of my face was gaunt and drooping. I decided to sleep it off. The next day I got up and did some painting. I noticed that my left hand was not working properly and I was still slurring my words. I was sleepy and felt like I had the flu.

I had no idea I had had a stroke. I still thought I was hung over or sick. I stayed at home until Grace returned five days later. She saw I wasn't well, so the next day we went to see our family doctor. She immediately sensed that I'd had a stroke and called to admit me to the hospital. I stayed there for three days and they confirmed that I had a "bleed" in the basal ganglia part of my brain, most likely resulting from high blood pressure, aggravated by an unusually high intake of alcohol.

I still wasn't completely convinced that I'd had a stroke. I had a monster-sized ego and thought I was bulletproof, so I was definitely in denial. . . . But it was a wake-up call. And I definitely wasn't all there. I called Grace the morning of the third day and told her that I had checked myself out and was at a girl's house around the corner, but I was actually still in the hospital and was completely disoriented.

Finally, I got the fact that I'd had a stroke. I still had a face droop, I was slurring my words, my left side was still uncoordinated, and I kept mixing up lines when I tried to read. They started me on some minor therapy to address these issues.

I felt much the same when I left the hospital as I did going in. My left leg dragged when I walked and it was not a pretty picture, but I still tried to talk Grace into allowing me to drive home. She adamantly refused. . . . I started outpatient therapy about a week after my release. The outpatient work was much more intensive and demanding than the little we did in the hospital. My speech therapist was very cute, and I worked extra hard with her.

My sight improved a bit, so I read and watched a little television. I started painting again about a week later. I was never that demanding of my left hand and arm, so the loss wasn't too much of an imposition, but I did need help with my pants and socks. I was very fatigued and took regular naps.

I was in decent shape before the stroke. I had started drinking more heavily in my mid-thirties, but my diet was decent and I was not overweight. I had been treating my high blood pressure for years and was taking medication, with check-ups every few months. I swam a few times a week in the warmer months and took walks. I had sleep apnea, and after my stroke I began using a CPAP machine for the condition. Before that I was only getting 75 percent of the oxygen I needed, which probably contributed to my stroke.

I guess I started coming to my senses, because I felt incredibly guilty about my behavior. My mother had warned me about my drinking, but I never heeded her advice. I was self-centered and selfish. She passed away a few months later, and her loss really hit me hard. I had heavy mood swings with bouts of uncontrolled crying that freaked out my friends. I might have lost a few, but my oldest friends have stayed with me. In fact, they think I'm more "normal" now—a less bionic version of my old self. I have upset my wife and made some of her family uncomfortable.

I used to be over the top in many ways; over-amplified. I was a cheerleader in high school and a singer. I was used to telling large crowds of people what to do. I used to have a booming voice that could clear a room. I was a lead singer in a rock band back in the sixties and used all the drugs of that era, which no doubt contributed to my oversized ego. I was very powerful and somewhat obnoxious. Since the stroke I have not been able to raise my voice to those levels, and now when

I sing a song longer than "Happy Birthday," I start to yawn.

I do not command a room like I used to, nor do I wish to. Two or three months after my stroke the doctor started me on an antidepressant called Cymbalta, which helped a lot, and I am still taking it.

After my stroke I taught drawing, painting, and architectural nomenclature for about a year at the college level. The school was a fifty-mile drive from home, and I fell asleep at the wheel on the highway one morning and crashed into a semi-truck. I had a severe injury to my leg, which made it painful to walk around. I ended up taking a semester off to heal, and when I returned they told me that enrollment had gone down and they had no place for me to teach. I found another teaching job closer to home three days a week.

I also had a job one day a week as an attendant at a marina where I had worked for a few years before my stroke. An employee who worked the other days told the supervisor that I had left the safe open, so he fired me. I know that I left the window open—and they had bars over them so no one could get in—but I didn't mean to leave the safe open, and I am not too sure that I even did that. They were concerned that I had come back too soon after my stroke, before I had all my wits about me. I was okay with leaving the job because I was bored. I am working on my résumé now and hope to find a new position soon.

Today I'm about thirty pounds overweight. My leg has pretty much healed, and I walk about a mile a day. My long-term planning is shot to hell. And my finances are in a horrible mess right now. I inherited a decent amount of money when my mother died, but I made some poor decisions and investments. I got calls from all kinds of leeches, and I was a pigeon for a number of get-rich-quick schemes. My stroke made me stupid. Fortunately we did save a little, and we mutually decided that Grace would take over our finances. On a more grounded level, I also manage a four-unit apartment house around the corner.

As a rule, I start to get ready for bed around 8:30 PM now, whereas I used to paint and draw until late—and I was very productive. These days, if I don't get something done by 8:30, then it's not getting done that day, because I'm too zapped. I still drink a glass or two of wine, but Grace is very much opposed, so occasionally I cut back for her.

My wife had Blue Cross from her school, and that was very helpful in terms of paying the hospital bill. I also had a long-term care policy, but in the long run I was too "healthy" to use it. The stroke did affect my ability to hold a quality job, so we have seen some financial hardship as a result of that.

I don't think I'd give back my stroke even if I could, unless I could retain all the life lessons I've learned. The stroke humbled me, and I have more empathy for people—disabled and otherwise. I've also had to park my ego and get a grip. I realize now that I can't do it all alone. I learned that I have to plan things out to get good results. I had to learn that people hold me accountable for what I say and that I can get into trouble for showing poor judgment. Until about two years ago, I was still oblivious to this. Before the stroke I *thought* that I was charming. I said what I wanted, but I've lost a few friends that way.

The stroke has made me a better person. I take things on a more personal level and hold them closer to my heart. I just couldn't understand all this before.

GRACE

Grace is Don's wife of twenty-five years. Like Don, Grace was an art teacher, and they've collaborated on many projects through the years.

I overheard some doctors talking after we knew that Don had suffered a stroke. They said he had some big problems and may not make it. When I realized that these were actually neurologists talking, I became very protective of Don. That first night he was panicking and didn't know how to handle this. He didn't know how to act. He asked me to get in bed with him, which I did, until the nurse said that I had to go. I kept thinking that I could help him and make everything all right.

He was not the same Don upon returning from the hospital, and he has never been the same Don since the stroke. His voice has become very quiet, where it used to be powerful and booming. The shape of his mouth is different. His eye droops when he gets tired, and he needs more sleep than he ever used to. He used to be a night owl, very creative and full of energy. His balance is also compromised; some days he struggles when getting into his jeans.

As he began to recover, his demeanor changed, and it became locked into this "new" Don. He slept a lot and cried a lot. I do, however, believe that Don will continue to get better. Doctors say that improvement wanes considerably after the first six months, but that's not what I've seen.

He's also become more self-centered. It's all about *me* and less about *we*, which is common with survivors—at least amongst the men. Sometimes I'm really put off and a little angry. As the caregiver, I have a huge amount of responsibility. Sometimes I forget about his condition and say, "Can't you be more sensitive and think about others?"

In our case, Don's made some very bad decisions and judgments, financially and emotionally. He got in the bathtub with a cast on his leg, without thinking about how he would get out. He started a kitchen remodel and had to stop. He gets the first part of the plan and then hits a "disconnect" before he sees it through to its conclusion. He mistakenly believes that everything will come out just fine. He also made some unsound investments that lost money, and I will probably have to go back to work to help out.

A lot of people will not ride in the car with him when he's driving now. I prefer to drive when we're together because I have fewer close calls. He hasn't had a bad accident, but his judgment is not what it used to be. I'm worried much of the time that I sit in the passenger seat, but I know that I shouldn't yell because it might distract him and make him less confident.

As a caregiver and loving spouse, we're supposed to accept "what is" and go on from there. Other spouses and therapists agree that it's difficult to see this behavior and completely accept it because it's so different from the behavior before the stroke. He's also less communicative, so it's hard to get to the truth and what's important. I know that's not a real positive outlook, but I am a forward-looking person and I keep hoping things will get better.

It's the emotional and cognitive difficulties that challenge me the most for sure. His impulse control is gone. He just goes headstrong into something, without much thought or planning—often with very costly results.

On some levels, I feel like I've lost a soul mate. There's a lot of him and a lot of me, but together we don't make a whole. There are moments and times when we are right there, like it used to be, but he *is* a different person. Sometimes it feels more like Don is my child than my partner, and that makes me cry. He doesn't want me to make the big decisions, but I have to be emotionally and financially responsible now.

There have been some funny moments, though, and we have kept our sense of humor. Don has done some very bizarre things that we could only laugh about. But he's cried much more than he's laughed. It's been hard to watch, and I've felt very bad for him.

We talk about these and other emotionally charged issues. I hope that I haven't painted a dark picture. We still have fun on occasion, and he can still make my heart zing. He is different, but I still love him dearly. I was very much inspired by the work he's done in therapy. I wanted him to work as hard as he could and I was very proud of him. And I still am. Some people refuse to do anything to help themselves or their spouses, but he's been great in that way.

Don thinks he's become more sensitive and empathetic since the stroke, but I'm not so sure. That may be the way he sees it, but I don't think he's shown that side to me. It's not that I don't love Don just as much as I did before the stroke, I just don't always see things the same way that he does. However, Don is right in one way: he's been so kind and caring and supportive of the people in his stroke support group. In that sense, he has been much more outgoing and less selfish than before his stroke.

I had to drag Don to the first few support group meetings. I needed help because I could not carry all of this on my own. I didn't realize how much I needed to hear from other people who were also going through this. Hearing and reading about what I should do is very different from actually meeting people who are going through the same things. It was a huge relief to see that I was not alone. It also showed me that it was going to be a long, rough road!

More importantly, the group has been quite nurturing for Don. It's also shown him that he has a lot to be thankful for and a lot to look forward to. He's actually driven group members to appointments and helped out where he could. We've also seen meaningful changes in other survivors in the group, which has helped Don feel better about his future.

Sometimes I become very concerned that Don could have another stroke. He will go into a manic state and get very intense. He goes headstrong into something and thinks of nothing else and won't slow down. I want him to exercise more and eat less. I didn't feel that way before his stroke.

I do believe that Don's stroke humbled him and made him a better person, and I have faith that he will continue along these lines and grow to regain many of his great qualities.

Sue & Sandy

Sue was fifty-six when she had her stroke; she is now sixty-two. Sue experienced one of the most life-changing and debilitating strokes I have encountered. She was an artist, full of energy and inspiration, when she was struck.

Sue

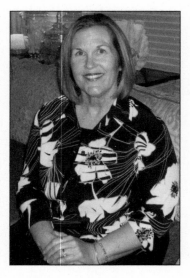

I started having severe headaches. I could hardly see, light was piercing and painful, and the discomfort was overwhelming, much more extreme than the average debilitating migraine. The headaches lasted about two hours. They'd stop for a while and then return. I was in good physical shape, and "stroke" never crossed my mind. I had no family history of stroke, but I checked in to the hospital for tests. We tried oxygen and injections, but nothing totally alleviated the pain. I was to be released after four days of inconclusive tests. When Sandy arrived he was confronted by a group of doctors telling him that they had to take me into surgery right away. The "bleed" apparently happened that morning, so at least I was in the right place at the right time.

I had lost my ability to speak, but I knew what had happened to my brain and my body. I was confused, and frustrated about being so confused. Then I passed out and do not remember anything until I woke after surgery.

A blood vessel had burst in my brain, causing inner-cranial bleeding. They removed a section of blood the size of two golf balls. I had suffered a hemorrhagic stroke, which may have been from vasculitis (an inflammation or swelling of the blood vessels). The doctors described the vessels as looking like little sausages.

The left side of my body was basically normal. I had right facial droop and the right side of my body—from head to toe—was shut down. I am right-handed, so this was traumatic. I couldn't talk or walk, and I saw things upside-down and sideways, out of focus.

I was mad and depressed. I was paralyzed. I could say yes and no, but often said yes when I meant no. I couldn't define up or down or left or right, and I still have difficulty with them now. I also had "locked-in" syndrome; lots of thoughts, but I could not express them. For the first couple of days I was heavily medicated, fighting confusion and struggling to get my bearings. I thought I was going to die and was fighting for my life. I never gave up hope because my will to live was strong. In my mind I felt that I could survive this.

Over two-and-a-half weeks I went from intensive care to critical care. I then spent two more weeks in a rehab center doing OT, ST, and PT, but my depression was the largest issue. I was started on antidepressants during that time. My inability to speak made communicating very difficult. I was fond of some of my nurses and disliked others, and it made a big difference in my treatment. Everything came slowly; there were no "aha" moments or breakthroughs.

I left in a wheelchair. I could not stand or use a walker and I could speak only a few words, but I was incredibly relieved to be going home. We moved my bed downstairs to Sandy's office on the main floor. We began assessing the day-to-day issues such as showering, brushing teeth, and all the other mundane things that you never think about when you are healthy. We had full-time caregivers to help us, and still do. I got better with every step, but it was very slow. The more I could do, the better I felt. I was very vulnerable, but I had a positive attitude within the confines of my limitations.

The outpatient program I attended was at a home that's affiliated with the hospital. I went five days a week starting about two months after my stroke, and I stayed with it for five months.

We would start at 9 AM doing OT, ST, and PT, followed by lunch, and then we'd repeat much the same thing in the afternoon, finishing up at 3 PM. This was work *and* socialization, so it was actually fun. The occupational therapist occasionally came back to our house to work with me and to help with everyday stuff. I was always exhausted when I left. I'd come home and collapse.

My short-term memory is definitely improving. I have two teachers who work with me on memory and numbers. We do vocabulary word exercises, and the math is coming along, albeit very slowly. I practice by repeating things and I play name games in my head to strengthen my abilities. . . . Acupuncture opened my neural pathways to recovery starting with my first session. It was nothing less than a miracle; I used to think it was voodoo, but now I do it every week.

It took two years to start reading. I could read line by line, but it was hard to find the next line. We used a piece of paper with a small rectangular box cut out to help me find the next line with less frustration. I took vision classes and had therapy for two years. My eyes were moving separately, and I needed to retrain them to move together as a pair. My vision is now very much improved. I retrained my brain to understand the images, and I slowly adapted to my new way of seeing, thinking, and processing information.

It took three or four months to start conversing. I think the acupuncture sessions did a tremendous amount of good. Speaking was the most important goal I had, and it took four-and-a-half years to speak this well.

I've been going to stroke support groups for two or three years, but went to an adult speech and support group before that. I am chairman of our book group and help select titles to read. The support groups are essential because we get the opportunity to learn and pass on knowledge. They are the only people to really understand what I've been going through.

As for painting, I am starting to get movement from my right side after four-and-a-half years of therapy, but I get so frustrated holding the paintbrush that the frustration is greater than the joy.

I walk on the treadmill twice a week. . . . I can walk with a cane, but I do spend most of my time in a wheelchair. I get a tremendous amount of support at PT and I get to socialize with people. I also take speech lessons and go to acupuncture sessions.

I can now appreciate how the stroke was one of the best things to happen to me. I have three daughters, and we have all become closer as a family as a result. I took too many things for granted, and now I have learned to appreciate the good things in my life. My daughters are also more understanding and are better people because of this experience. . . . I've been able to overcome almost all obstacles; and I feel there is no end to what I can accomplish. It's now been seven years since my stroke and I can honestly say, against everyone's prognostication, I continue to improve and feel better every day! My mind is clearer and my family has rallied round me.

SANDY

You have to understand that Sue is a highly motivated woman. If you give her a goal, she will achieve it, and then some. Her attitude is: I'm doing this, and if I have to walk through a wall, I will. The rehabilitation staff at the hospital thought she was too far gone to make much of an improvement, but she proved them all wrong. They said that most improvement begins to diminish after one to two years, but at four-and-a-half years she is still making impressive strides, and we don't see that stopping anytime soon. . . .

The apraxia—the inability to carry out purposeful movements, despite having the desire and the physical ability—and aphasia present a two-fold challenge. Sue can walk at home using a cane with little problem, but her apraxia, which is quite severe, affects her ability to adjust to new places. The aphasia affects her vision, so she may be able to enter an unfamiliar room, but the lines in a carpet will look like they are moving, which throws off her balance and bearing. And if there's an object in the way of her stride, she can't tell if the object is flat or not. . . .

And the apraxia prevents her from working well enough with her left hand to satisfy her artistic tastes. She does basic things such as eating (with a special plate that has sides so she can push the food onto a spoon), and she can pour herself a drink from a can, but she cannot perform complex movements, such as tying her shoes.

The whole process has made me a better person. In our household, prior to the stroke, I took care of the business and Susie took care of everything else, including plumbing and house repairs. Now I've had to learn these other tasks. I think I've shocked my daughters by proving I can use a hammer, when they assumed—perhaps quite accurately—that I didn't know which end was up.

It's changed my life. I think the depression accompanying a stroke applies to the spouse, too, even though mine was nothing like Sue's. I was extremely independent prior to the stroke, and Susie allowed me that independence in our marriage. Now I have to concern myself with everything, whereas before my job was to make sure funds were rolling in and to involve myself with the kids when needed. It's all-consuming. But things are getting back to some version of the past, after four-and-a-half years.

I've had my own business for the last thirty years, and I work at home, so I was able to be present during this whole period. I'm an agent for toy inventors. I used to go to Japan five or six times a year, and I now go four times. We have caregivers who we love and trust, and they are invaluable.

Our daughters live locally, and they have all been an unbelievably positive support. They have learned about appreciating life and recognizing what can happen and how to handle change. Watching Susie fight through this thing has provided wonderful life lessons for them.

PART THREE

GLOSSARY AND RESOURCES

GLOSSARY

aphasia
Aphasia is a loss of the ability to produce and/or comprehend language. Depending on the area and extent of the damage, someone suffering from aphasia may be able to speak but not write, or vice versa. It is not, however, an indication of intelligence.

apraxia
Apraxia is a neurological disorder characterized by loss of the ability to execute or carry out learned purposeful movements (such as walking), despite having the desire and the physical ability to perform the movements.

AVM
Arteriovenous malformation (AVM) is an abnormal connection between veins and arteries, usually congenital. This pathology is widely known because of its occurrence in the central nervous system, but can appear in any location.

ASD
Atrial septal defect (ASD) is a form of congenital heart defect that enables blood flow between the left and right atria via the interatrial septum. The interatrial septum is the tissue that divides the right and left atria. Without this septum, or if there is a defect in this septum, it is possible for blood to travel from the left side of the heart to the right side of the heart, or vice versa.

basal ganglia
The basal ganglia (or basal nuclei) are a group of nuclei (neuron clusters) in the brain interconnected with the cerebral

cortex, thalamus and brainstem. This is the area of the brain that felled a few of our survivors.

brain stem

The brain stem is the lower part of the brain, adjoining and structurally continuous with the spinal cord. The brain stem provides the main motor and sensory innervation (activity) to the face and neck via the cranial nerves. Though small, this is an extremely important part of the brain as the nerve connections of the motor and sensory systems from the main part of the brain to the rest of the body pass through the brain stem.

cardiothoracic surgery

Cardiothoracic surgery is the field of medicine involved in surgical treatment of diseases affecting organs inside the thorax (chest), treatment of conditions of the heart and lungs.

carotid artery

In human anatomy, the common carotid artery is an artery that supplies the head and neck with oxygenated blood.

coumadin (warfarin)

Warfarin (also known under the brand names Coumadin, Jantoven, Marevan, and Waran) is an anticoagulant. A few years after its introduction, warfarin was found to be effective and relatively safe for preventing thrombosis and embolism (abnormal formation and migration of blood clots) in many disorders. Usually the drug of choice for stroke patients and those with heart ailments after stent surgery.

craniotomy

A craniotomy is a surgical operation in which part of the skull, called a bone flap, is removed in order to access the brain.

cryptogenic stroke
A cryptogenic stroke is a stroke in which the true cause cannot be determined.

CT
Computed tomography, also referred to as a "CAT Scan." It is used to image blood flow and blockages, such as dissected arteries and blood clots. It is different than an MRI.

CVST
Cerebral venous sinus thrombosis (CVST) is a rare form of stroke that results from thrombosis (a blood clot) of the dural venous sinuses, which drain blood from the brain. Symptoms may include headache, abnormal vision, any of the symptoms of stroke such as weakness of the face and limbs on one side of the body, and seizures.

echocardiogram
An echocardiogram, often referred to in the medical community as a cardiac ECHO or simply an ECHO, is a sonogram of the heart. Also known as a cardiac ultrasound, it uses standard ultrasound techniques to image two-dimensional slices of the heart. The latest ultrasound systems now employ 3D real-time imaging.

EKG
An electrocardiogram (ECG or EKG) is a recording of the electrical activity of the heart over time produced by an electrocardiograph, usually in a noninvasive recording via skin electrodes.

ENT
ENT is the abbreviation for an ear, nose, and throat specialist.

EMT
Emergency medical technician, also called ambulance technicians. EMTs respond to emergency calls, perform certain medical procedures, and transport patients to the hospital.

F.A.S.T.
The signs of stroke:

FACE – Ask the person to smile. Does one side of the face droop?
ARMS – Ask the person to raise both arms. Does one arm drift downward?
SPEECH – Ask the person to repeat a simple sentence (e.g. "It's sunny today."). Are the words slurred? Can the person repeat the sentence correctly?
TIME – If the person shows any symptoms, time is important. Call 911 immediately.

hemorrhagic stroke
Bleeding, technically known as hemorrhaging, is the loss of blood or blood escape from the circulatory system. Bleeding can occur internally, where blood leaks from blood vessels inside the body or externally.

heparin
This medication is an anticoagulant that prevents the blood from clotting. It is used to prevent and treat venous thrombosis, pulmonary embolism, and other conditions of blood clotting. (www.medicinenet.com)

interventional cardiology
Interventional cardiology is a branch of the medical specialty of cardiology that deals specifically with the catheter-based treatment of structural heart diseases. (PFO repair, etc.)

interventional radiology
Interventional radiology (abbreviated IR or sometimes VIR for vascular and interventional radiology) is a subspecialty of radiology in which minimally invasive procedures are performed using image guidance.

ischemic (is-skeem-ic) stroke

Occurs when an artery to the brain is blocked. The brain depends on its arteries to bring fresh blood from the heart and lungs. The blood carries oxygen and nutrients to the brain and takes away carbon dioxide and cellular waste. If an artery is blocked, the brain cells cannot make enough energy and will eventually stop working. If the artery remains blocked for more than a few minutes, the brain cells may die. This is why immediate medical treatment is absolutely critical. (www.strokecenter.org)

MRI

Magnetic resonance imaging (MRI), or nuclear magnetic resonance imaging (NMRI), is primarily a medical imaging technique most commonly used in radiology to visualize the internal structure and function of the body. In the case of stroke victims, it is used to view clots in the brain. MRI provides much greater contrast between the different soft tissues of the body than computed tomography (CT) does.

PFO

PFO (Patent foramen ovale) is the term for the condition known as a "hole in the heart." The prevalence of PFO is about 25 percent in the general population. In patients who have stroke of unknown cause (cryptogenic stroke), the prevalence of PFO increases to about 40 percent. This is especially true in patients who have had a stroke at age less than 55 years. (A PFO can be repaired, as it was on a number of the stroke survivors in our interviews.) (www.my.clevelandclinic.org)

Plavix (clopidogrel)

Clopidogrel is an oral antiplatelet agent to inhibit blood clots in coronary artery disease, peripheral vascular disease, and cerebrovascular disease. It is marketed under the trade name Plavix.

TCD

Transcranial Doppler (TCD) is a test that measures the velocity of blood-flow through the brain's blood vessels.

TIA

A transient ischemic attack (TIA), often referred to as "mini stroke," is caused by the changes in the blood supply to a particular area of the brain, resulting in brief neurologic dysfunction that persists, by definition, for less than 24 hours; if symptoms persist, then it is categorized as a stroke. The most frequent symptoms include temporary loss of vision, difficulty speaking, weakness on one side of the body, and numbness or tingling usually confined to one side of the body.

TEE

Transesophageal Echocardiogram or TEE is an echocardiogram (often called an "echo"), a graphic outline of the heart's movement, valves and chambers. During the TEE test, an ultrasound transducer provides pictures of the heart's valves and chambers and helps the physician evaluate the pumping action of the heart. The endoscope is placed into your mouth and passed into your esophagus (the "food pipe" leading from your mouth into your stomach) to provide a close look at your heart's valves and chambers without interference from the ribs or lungs. (my.clevelandclinic.org)

TEE is often combined with Doppler ultrasound and color Doppler to evaluate blood flow across the heart's valves. TEE is often used when the results from standard echo studies were not sufficient or when your doctor wants a closer look at your heart.

TPA

TPA (plasminogen activator) is a "clot-busting drug." The drug can dissolve blood clots and it is the only drug approved by the FDA for the acute treatment of ischemic stroke. However, to be effective, it must be given within a few hours after symptoms begin. (American Heart.org)

Valsalva maneuver
The Valsalva maneuver is performed by forcibly exhaling against a closed airway. This test can be used to identify the presence of a hole in the heart. This process was used on a few of our survivors.

vasculitis
Vasculitis is an inflammation of the blood vessels. Also called angiitis, vasculitis causes changes in the walls of your blood vessels, including thickening, weakening, narrowing and scarring. (www.mayoclinic.com)

vertebral artery
Inside the skull, the two vertebral arteries join up to form the basilar artery at the base of the medulla oblongata. The basilar artery is the main blood supply to the brainstem and connects to the Circle of Willis to potentially supply the rest of the brain if there is compromise to one of the carotids.

Exercises for Therapy:
Remember to switch hands and legs whenever possible. Try to do each process with both sides of the body to create equality, even if it's nearly impossible at the beginning of each pursuit. Be sure to check with your doctors and therapists to certify that these exercises will be safe for you to do.

- Chinese Balls for finger and hand dexterity
- Crumbling newspaper into a ball with one hand, also for finger and hand control
- Digi-Flex to strengthen hand and fingers
- Twirling or spinning a cell phone to help with hand control; this can be done at home or on the run.
- Snapping your fingers until you can get an audible "snap" that matches your better hand
- Therapy Putty to strengthen fingers
- Unscrewing bottle tops with the weak hand . . . I used to naturally hold a bottle in my left hand and unscrew

the top with my right. I now hold the bottle in my right hand and use my gimpy left hand to unscrew the top. Finger twirling and stretching to make them feel part of your body

- Picking stones out of a bowl of sand, rice, or bird seed to improve dexterity and control
- Washing dishes to increase awareness and strength: Helps you re-learn how to hold a glass. Once you can wash dishes with control, switch hands and hold the glass or dish with your "off hand" to become skilled on both sides. This may take weeks or months.
- Folding clothing helps with cognitive and physical ability
- Clapping hands together and against your leg
- Folding paper into squares to improve articulation and control
- Bouncing a ball and catching it with each hand, rotating after each bounce
  o Try the same bounce and catch while walking
- Folding paper into squares

To learn more about stroke, visit the following websites:

American Stroke Association – www.strokeassociation.org

American Heart Association – www.americanheart.org

Stroke Center – www.strokecenter.org/patients/stats.htm

U.S. Stroke Statistics

- Stroke remains the third leading cause of death, behind heart disease and cancer.
- The ideal treatment window for most strokes is within the first three hours, and only 3-5 % of patients make it to the hospital in time for treatment. Most people don't know the signs of stroke. A recent survey showed that

people fear having a stroke more than dying because of the disability they may have. Stroke is the leading cause of serious, long-term disability in the United States. In 1999, about 1,100,000 Americans reported difficulties with daily living because of a stroke.

- Each year, about 700,000 people suffer a stroke. About 500,000 of these are first attacks, and 200,000 are recurrent attacks. Stroke killed 275,000 people in 2002 and accounted for about 1 of 16 deaths in the United States. 28% of people who suffer a stroke in a given year are under the age 65. Compared with white males 45 to 54 years old, African American males in the same age group have a three-fold greater risk of ischemic stroke. About 50% of stroke deaths in 2003 occurred out of the hospital. On average, someone in the United States suffers a stroke every 45 seconds; every 3 to 4 minutes, someone dies of a stroke. About 4.7 million stroke survivors (2.3 million men, 2.4 million women) are alive today. Among persons 45 to 64 years old, 8-12% of ischemic strokes and 37-38% of hemorrhagic strokes result in death within 30 days. Quitting smoking reduces your stroke risk to that of a non-smoker in five years. Sickle cell disease is the most important cause of ischemic stroke among African American children. Within a year, up to 25% of people who have had a transient ischemic attack will die. This percentage is higher among people 65 and older.

Want Steve Boorstein to speak at your book club, support group, or next event?

Email steve@survivingstroke.com